The management of nutrition in major emergencies

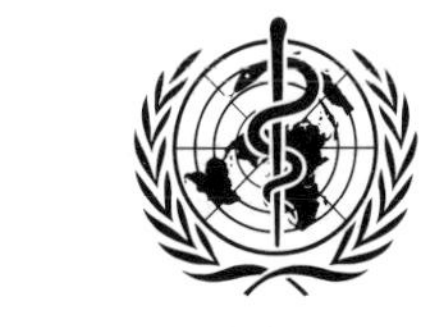

World Health Organization
Geneva
2000

WHO Library Cataloguing-in-Publication Data

The Management of nutrition in major emergencies.
1.Emergency feeding 2.Nutritional requirements 3.Nutritional status 4.Nutrition disorders — prevention and control 5.Communicable disease control 6.Emergencies 7.Manuals

ISBN 92 4 154520 8 (NLM classification: QU 145)

Designed by WHO Graphics
Typeset in Hong Kong
Printed in Malta
97/11724 — Best-Set/Interprint — 7500

Contents

Preface

This manual is intended to help health, nutrition, and other professionals involved in the management of major emergencies with a nutritional component, whether at local, national, or international level. By improving understanding among the health professionals and intersectoral personnel who are collectively responsible for ensuring adequate nutrition in emergency-affected populations, the manual should promote coordinated and effective action.

All major emergencies, by definition, threaten human life and public health. They often result in food shortages, impair or jeopardize the nutritional status of a community, and cause excess mortality in all age groups. Nutrition is therefore a key public health concern in emergency management. Accordingly, this manual deals with the following topics: initial nutritional assessments; identifying the risk or presence of various forms of malnutrition; calculating food needs and, where necessary, ensuring generalized or selective food distribution; treating malnutrition and preventing the occurrence of nutritional deficiencies; monitoring the nutritional status and the food availability in households; and preventing and controlling nutrition-related and food-borne communicable diseases.

The occurrence of both natural and man-made emergencies has risen dramatically in recent years, with a parallel growth in the numbers of stricken communities, refugees, and internally displaced persons. The International Conference on Nutrition, convened by FAO and WHO in 1992, devoted much time to the nutrition of refugees, and displaced and war-affected populations — "the world's most malnourished nation". The *World Declaration and Plan of Action for Nutrition,*[1] signed by 159 ministerial representatives and the then European Economic Community, urged governments to provide sustainable assistance to these people and to ensure their nutritional well-being. Part 6 of the World Plan of Action (Caring for the socio-economically deprived and nutritionally vulnerable) states in Article 37:

> "Among refugees and displaced populations, high rates of malnutrition and micronutrient deficiencies associated with high rates of mortality continue to occur. The magnitude of the problem has grown over the last decade. Increased political commitment to and accountability for the protection and promotion of the nutritional well-being of refugees, displaced populations, those under occupation, prisoners of war and other affected groups are urgently required in accordance with international humani-

[1] *World Declaration and Plan of Action for Nutrition, Rome, December 1992.* Geneva, World Health Organization, 1992 (unpublished document ICN/92/2).

tarian law. Governments, in collaboration with the international community, should:

(a) Provide sustainable assistance to refugees and displaced persons and work to monitor their nutritional well-being, giving high priority to the control of diseases and to the prevention of malnutrition and outbreaks of micronutrient deficiency disease. Wherever feasible such assistance should encourage their ability to support themselves rather than increase their dependence on external assistance. The food provided should be nutritionally adequate and safe.

(b) Identify, within civilian populations situated in zones of conflict, refugee and displaced populations and groups needing special care including the disabled, the elderly, children, mothers and other nutritionally vulnerable groups in order to provide for their special needs."

In response to the World Declaration, almost all countries have developed, or are developing, a national plan of action for nutrition, which should include action for preparedness and capacity-building for management of nutrition in emergencies.

While awareness of the risk and burden of malnutrition in emergency situations has grown, there have also been many advances in knowledge in the fields of nutrition, of emergency preparedness and response, and of the interrelations between disasters and development, and consequent improvements in practice. This manual deals primarily with the nutritional aspects of emergency relief, but it also reflects these new approaches to management, preparedness, prevention, and rehabilitation. This new knowledge has already been put to extensive use in various emergency situations, such as the severe crop failures in southern Africa in the early 1990s; thanks to better management of generalized food distribution and other supportive health measures there were very few surplus deaths and no widespread severe undernutrition.

It is important that nutrition-related interventions be viewed and undertaken as an integral part of a comprehensive approach to emergency management in affected areas. This also implies the inclusion of nutrition in overall emergency preparedness. It is a regrettable fact that, up to now, much of the action in emergency situations has been taken by external agencies, often by-passing national nutritional institutions. This is attributable partly to lack of adequate national resources but also to inadequate preparedness. The 1978 WHO monograph *The management of nutritional emergencies in large populations*, together with the World Declaration and Plan of Action, provided valuable inspiration and background material for the present manual. This manual, and the learning modules and human resource development programmes to be derived from it, should help to reinforce national capacities and enable national authorities, institutions, and nutrition programmes in particular, to ensure adequate management of nutrition in emergencies. The guidelines should be equally valuable to any organizations cooperating with the government in the management of an emergency.

One important lesson drawn from the experiences since publication of the 1978 monograph is that emergency management is a multisectoral and institutional venture: it cannot be the domain only of the national or local government or of military authorities. Ministries and departments of local government, health, agriculture, environment, welfare, finance, trade, transport, communications, and public works need to plan and work together for emergency prevention, preparedness and response, and rehabilitation.

A second lesson has been that disasters do not occur in a vacuum: they originate from disturbances of the physical, social, or economic milieu, and they can have long-term consequences for nutrition and development itself. Malnutrition may be the primary feature of an emergency, as in drought or flood with subsequent famine, or may be its painful consequence, as in war, mass displacement, or economic disaster. Either way, nutritional considerations are an inescapable element of any major emergency. Particular understanding and efforts are essential to ensure adequate nutrition both in the relief phase and during the subsequent rehabilitation and development phases.

Drought is often the proximate cause of food shortage. However, it is rarely the sole, or even the basic, cause. Emergency preparedness must deal with the deeper causes and, when needed, with the chain of results following food shortage. The consequences of cyclic ("normal") decreases in rainfall may be exacerbated by poor management of land and environment, demographic pressures, inadequate or inappropriate farming technologies, and poor infrastructure, leading to periodic food shortages. Economic constraints at the local, national, and international (trade) levels can all aggravate a marginal food situation. The poorest countries often have inadequate services and safety nets to cope with severe recurrent or periodic stress. Loss of production, however, does not only produce food shortages. Employment and purchasing power are also lost, trade and marketing systems break down, and prices increase dramatically; thus poor urban people are affected, as well as farming populations. Shortage of water may cause the death of livestock, increase the risk of diarrhoeal disease, and even affect the productivity of local industries and the production of energy. Soil structure, vegetation, and wildlife can all be seriously and even irreversibly affected.

Survival strategies at family and community level often include selling basic assets, migration, and disruption of households. Parents are likely to be too busy to take their children regularly to health clinics unless the clinics are nearby. Such widespread poverty, bringing physical, mental, social, and economic hardship, will accentuate vulnerability to nutritional deficiencies. The environment and socioeconomic fabric of an entire country or region can suffer a prolonged set-back.

This brief analysis highlights the need to develop emergency preparedness and management capacities, and so reduce the vulnerability of the population and mitigate the consequences of the crisis. Preparedness is crucial to the community's survival and continuing development.

It is beyond the scope of this book to deal in detail with food security, emergency preparedness, and rehabilitation. The initial rapid-assessment phase — when famine or risk of famine is suspected — is dealt with in another WHO manual, *Rapid health assessment protocols for emergencies* (1999). Rapid health assessment is likely to be the first and immediate action required in an existing emergency situation, and may or may not involve nutrition specialists. The multisectoral and interdisciplinary (health) process for emergency preparedness is dealt with in the WHO publication *Community emergency preparedness: a manual for managers and policy-makers* (1999). Only the broad lines of approach to management in the rehabilitation and development phases are given in this manual, mainly in Chapter 7.

A third lesson learned since the 1978 monograph is that ensuring adequate nutrition in emergencies compels a holistic and proactive approach, which implies more than food distribution and protection of health. Intersectoral and comprehensive action is called for in the areas of environment, population, economic and human development, land and water management, food production and trade, services, human rights, governance, empowerment, and growth of the civil society. The health sector has a precise role to play in all these areas, providing education, advocacy, and technical expertise to ensure vulnerability reduction and preparedness for appropriate nutrition-related relief, treatment and prevention of malnutrition, and ultimately promotion of nutrition in the context of broader health, community rehabilitation, and development policy.

For emergency relief to be effective, preparedness is vital. A country with a strong preparedness system will be ready to respond to emergencies effectively and efficiently, allowing the normal development processes to be resumed as rapidly as possible. Effective handling of an emergency requires countries to establish mechanisms that can provide early warning of impending difficulty and deal proactively with the needs (rather than simply rely on external agencies to provide relief activities and food). This manual identifies the basic nutritional needs and hazards of an emergency situation and the national programmes required to safeguard the nutrition of the population.

If governments do not take these steps in advance it will prove near-impossible to break the vicious cycle of poverty, undernutrition, and underdevelopment at any level of society. Ecosystems will be increasingly degraded, mass movements of people will continue. The demand for short-term relief will continue to grow, fostering dependency and a stop-gap approach to a crisis that has deep-rooted, but preventable, causes.

Experience gained since publication of the 1978 monograph has also shown that the primary responsibility for disaster/emergency management must rest with national governments, in a framework of decentralization. For policies and plans to be effective, the authority and resources for their implementation should be decentralized to sub-national levels. International, bilateral, and nongovernmental organizations and the private sector should complement and support the national goals and mechanisms of emergency preparedness and management. When disaster strikes and relief is needed, these groups should accept coordination by the national authorities. Where the government is not in control, external agencies for emergency relief coordination may take temporary responsibility for essential operations, but all special humanitarian assistance programmes should respect the primary need for building or rebuilding national capacities for managing both the relief phase and the transition to rehabilitation and development phases.

A final lesson is that communities and families themselves have often developed some coping strategies, particularly if they have been involved previously in emergencies. The goal of emergency preparedness and response is essentially to enhance this self-help capacity, as well as to ensure all the support necessary to enable each community to manage the health, food, and nutrition situation adequately.

As regards nutrition, this approach offers a particular challenge. Very often countries have a national nutrition unit and programme, but lack nutrition personnel at district and lower levels. General health, agriculture, and administrative personnel therefore need reinforcement of their technical knowledge and skills if they are to respond appropriately and meet the nutritional needs. Human resource development programmes at all levels are thus crucial in most emergency-prone countries and should be given the highest priority for immediate action. It is also important to inculcate and facilitate the habit of working together across sectoral boundaries.

In brief, nutrition is a key component of emergency preparedness and response. Hunger and starvation have immediate health, humanitarian, and political dimensions. In an emergency, a ministry of health will be called on to respond to daily queries about the affected populations and their needs, to dissipate rumours, to mobilize support, and to undertake powerful advocacy. Ideally, the ministry should be aware of, and be able to coordinate and facilitate, the work of all concerned with nutrition in emergencies, including international partners.

The nutrition section of a health ministry, in close coordination with the section responsible for interdisciplinary emergency management, should have the capacity and structure of a highly organized technical and managerial unit, able to carry out functions such as those listed in the box on the following page.

Since the essential purpose of this manual is to help build national capacity for managing emergencies, and this implies human resource development within the country, Annex 9 of this manual provides a framework for a human resource development programme for the management of nutrition in emergencies, in the form of appropriate general, intermediate and specific objectives. These would have to be adapted to the national circumstances and would then become the basis for defining the content of a training course, most of the material for which is covered in this manual.

Acknowledgements

A special debt of gratitude is owed to the following individuals who contributed chapters and/or made other significant textual inputs to the development of this manual: Kenneth V. Bailey, Angela Berry, Graeme A. Clugston, Bruno de Benoist, Danielle Deboutte, Olivier Fontaine, Susan Peele Morris, Philip Nieburg, Ron Ockwell, Clare Schofield, and Zita Weise Prinzo.

WHO is also grateful to the following people for reviewing the manuscript at different stages and providing valuable comments: Anne Ashworth, David Alnwick, Rita Bhatia, Sarah Ballance, Mercedes de Onis, Claude de Ville de Goyet, Mohammed Dualeh, Natalie Domieson, Ellen Edwards-Wasserman, Anna Ferro-Luzzi, Michael Gurney, Stephen Hansch, Ailsa Holloway, Philip James, Wolf Keller, Stephen Lwanga, John Mason, Julia Stuckey, Michael Teihades, Michael Toole, and Anna Verster.

Many helpful inputs were provided by the staff of various WHO departments on a range of nutrition, health, emergency, and logistic issues such as those relating to diarrhoeal disease, environmental health, food safety, immunization, and malaria. Grateful acknowledgement is therefore made to the Departments of Emergency and Humanitarian Action, Nutrition for Health and Development, Child and Adolescent Health, Protection of the Human Environment, and Vaccines and Other Biologicals, and to nutrition staff in the WHO regional offices. WHO is also grateful for the comments provided by the ACC/SCN (United Nations Administrative Committee on Coordination/Sub-committee on Nutrition) Ad Hoc Working Group on Nutrition of Refugees and Displaced People.

WHO wishes to thank the International Federation of Red Cross and Red Crescent Societies (IFRC), the Office of the United Nations High Commissioner for Refugees (UNHCR), and the World Food Programme (WFP) for their financial support for the development and publication of this manual.

Main functions of a national nutrition programme in emergencies

- Identifying, in health and other information systems, data, indicators and sources for nutritional surveillance and early warning.
- Collecting and storing baseline data, analysing and disseminating relevant information, for purposes of policy-making, strategic planning, advocacy, and public awareness and participation.
- Defining strategies, programmes, technical standards, guidelines, and procedures (including food ration and distribution systems, newsletters/bulletins, lists of nutrition resource persons in the area) for nutritional and food surveillance, generalized, selective, and therapeutic feeding programmes, and micronutrient fortification or supplementation.
- Organizing rapid assessments to determine the presence and extent of nutritional emergencies, and full assessments of nutritional status in valid samples of children and adults.
- Developing continuing surveillance of nutritional status in emergency-affected areas, including monitoring the adequacy of food distribution systems and the impact of interventions, and contributing to the building and interpretation of databases on food availability and its adequacy, food stocks, logistic systems, food control systems, etc.
- Ensuring that appropriate therapeutic management is provided for severely malnourished individuals.
- Developing institutional and human capacities and learning materials for in-service training of nutritionists and other health and administrative staff, including those responsible for food distribution, handling, preparation, etc., and for therapeutic feeding, and for strengthening training curricula on nutrition in emergencies for all categories of health personnel.
- Liaising with the emergency coordination cell and other health units and programmes, exchanging information and plans, integrating nutrition activities in primary health care, and coordinating with the nutrition-related components of other programmes and/or activities (e.g. immunization, control of diarrhoeal diseases, maternal and child health, and environmental health services including food safety).
- Liaising, through the emergency coordination cell, with other relevant ministries (e.g. local government, agriculture, social welfare, community development, commerce, finance, public works), as well as with relief and development agencies, for information and advocacy concerning nutritional needs, and to seek their technical, material, and/or financial support for intersectoral plans and operations, including appropriate local food production, processing, and marketing.
- Participating in the activities of national coordination committees for food security, food distribution, monitoring and nutrition risk-mapping, advocacy, and resource-mobilization.

CHAPTER 1

Meeting nutritional requirements

In major emergencies, one of the most urgently needed actions to prevent death and illness caused by malnutrition is to ensure adequate provision and intake of food. Basic energy and protein requirements are the primary concern, but micronutrient and other specific nutrient needs must also be met if blindness, disability, and death are to be avoided.

Assessment of the nutritional requirements of the population is a fundamental management tool for calculating food needs, monitoring the adequacy of food access and intake, and ensuring adequate food procurement.

Since the energy and protein requirements of the population are usually unknown to begin with, a mean daily per capita intake of 2100 $kcal_{th}$ and 46 g of protein is recommended (for a developing country profile). Mean daily intakes of micronutrients and other specific nutrients are also recommended in this chapter. Once population and environmental characteristics are known and can be applied, more accurate calculations of population nutrient requirements can be made.

The monitoring of food intakes in the affected community is essential, to enable national authorities both to assess the adequacy of food distribution and to determine when it may be safely decreased and ultimately terminated.

Meeting nutritional requirements in emergency situations — principles

Malnutrition in one or more of its various forms frequently characterizes emergency situations, both natural and man-made. Ensuring that the food and nutrition needs of disaster-stricken populations, refugees, or internally displaced people are adequately met is often the principal component of the humanitarian, logistic, management, and financial response to an emergency. When the nutritional needs of a population — or population subgroup — are not completely met, some form of malnutrition soon emerges, usually among the most helpless or vulnerable individuals. The results are underweight children, anaemic mothers, marasmic babies, scurvy, beriberi, pellagra, vitamin A deficiency blindness, and other deficiency syndromes.

If the nutritional requirements of individuals, groups, and populations are to be met, the average daily intake of each nutrient needs to be sufficient to:

- cover losses of each nutrient
- take account of nutrient interactions in the diet
- take account of environmental conditions
- maintain physical size, growth, pregnancy, lactation
- maintain activity, including economically necessary and socially desirable activity.

Knowledge of human nutritional requirements is essential in the management of nutritional emergencies for three important and closely linked purposes:

- assessing the food needs of particular individuals, families, and vulnerable groups and of the population as a whole;
- monitoring the adequacy of nutrient intake in these groups;
- ensuring that food procurement for general rations, supplementary feeding, therapeutic feeding, etc. is sufficient to meet the nutritional needs of all.

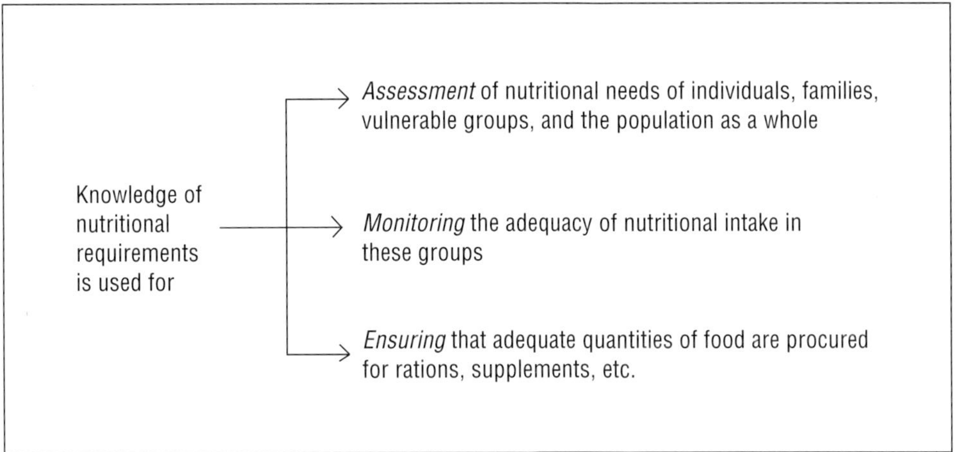

It is also essential to identify the most vulnerable groups in the population, which generally include:

- pregnant and lactating women, because they have additional nutrient needs;
- infants and young children, who may not be able to consume or digest the foods provided, and who are particularly prone to malnutrition because of their proportionately high nutritional requirements;
- families or individuals whose needs may not be fully met by a particular ration distribution system, especially in the cases of families with large numbers of adults, and of elderly single adults, widows, and widowers.

Meeting energy and protein requirements

In famines and other emergencies involving food shortages and affecting large populations, one of the most immediate aims of relief efforts is to prevent death and illness caused by malnutrition and infectious disease. The question of how much food is needed to feed a disaster-stricken population must be urgently addressed.

The first concern is to ensure that energy and protein requirements are met. Little may be known about the target population except the number of persons affected, and a single guideline for meeting average energy and protein requirements can then be extremely useful, facilitating decisions about the immediate procurement of food for use as emergency rations.

In these circumstances, the estimated average daily per capita energy requirement for a typical developing country population is 2070 $kcal_{th}$; a rounded-up

Daily energy requirements and safe protein intake

The estimated mean daily per capita energy requirement of 2070 $kcal_{th}$, rounded up to 2100 $kcal_{th}$, is based on WHO Technical Report No. 724 (*Energy and protein requirements. Report of a Joint FAO/WHO/UNU Expert Consultation*), published in 1985, and on the following assumptions:

- the age/sex distribution of the population is characteristic of developing countries;
- the mean heights of adult men and women are 169 cm and 155 cm, respectively, which approximate values in sub-Saharan Africa;
- the weights of adults are such that body mass index (BMI) is between 20 and 22;
- physical activity is light;
- all infants are breast-fed from birth to 6 months, and half the infants of 6–11 months are still breast-feeding and deriving half their energy and protein needs from breast milk.

Safe daily protein intake, from an average mixed diet of cereals, pulses, and vegetables, is estimated to be 46 g.

value of 2100 $kcal_{th}$ is suggested.[1,2] The average safe protein intake per person per day is 46 g of mixed-diet protein, where the mixed diet is composed of cereal, pulses, and vegetables. For practical purposes, these guidelines may be used for most populations until more population-specific information becomes available.

Mean daily per capita requirements may vary from population to population, but the mean daily energy requirement is usually between 1900 and 2300 $kcal_{th}$. The requirements are influenced by a number of population and environmental factors, including the following, which should be assessed and taken into account as soon as possible, to ensure that energy and protein requirements can be met:

- age and sex composition of the population
- mean adult heights and weights (men and women)
- physical activity levels
- environmental temperatures
- malnutrition and ill-health
- food security.

Annex 1 details age- and sex-specific daily energy and protein requirements, and population characteristics used in their calculation. It also shows the additional energy needed for moderate or heavy activity (as in populations walking long distances or engaged in manual labour) and in cold environments.

If average daily energy intake falls below the calculated mean requirement taking account of these population and environmental factors, the basic nutritional needs of a significant part of the population are unlikely to be met. This will then increase the risk of continuing malnutrition and ill-health, especially in vulnerable groups such as infants and young children and pregnant women. It may also delay the recovery time for a population already debilitated by prolonged food deprivation. When a diet does not provide enough energy, the body will begin to consume for energy purposes the protein that it needs for growth and repair. If based on a cereal/pulse/vegetable mixture, most diets that meet energy needs will also provide adequate quantities of protein.

Fat or oil is also a significant dietary component of the ration. It enhances palatability and provides energy in a concentrated form (see Annex 2). To cover the requirements for certain essential fatty acids, it is recommended that fats/oils provide at least 15% of the total energy intake of adults (but 20% for women of reproductive age) and 30–40% for children up to 2 years of age. Overall, it is recommended that fats/oils should comprise 17–20% of the ration, although

[1] This is consistent with the value of 2100 $kcal_{th}$ recommended by Committee on Nutrition, National Academy of Sciences, and published in: *Estimated mean per capita energy requirements for planning emergency food aid rations*. Washington, DC, National Academy Press, 1995.

[2] In the field of nutrition it is still common for energy requirements to be quoted in calories — or, more correctly, thermochemical calories (cal_{th}). The SI unit of energy is in fact the **joule**, and the relationship between the two units is 1 $kcal_{th}$ = 4.18 kJ. Thus, the estimated daily per capita energy requirement of 2100 $kcal_{th}$ = 8.78 MJ.

saturated fatty acids (found in animal fats and some vegetable oils) should not provide more than 10% of dietary energy.[1]

Meeting micronutrient and other specific nutrient requirements

Nutritional emergencies may be characterized not only by protein–energy malnutrition, wasting, and growth failure but also by a variety of micronutrient (mineral and vitamin) deficiencies, some of which lead to blindness, disability, paralysis, and death. Prevention of these deficiencies should be a further consideration in determining the food requirements. Chapter 2 outlines the main symptoms and signs of these conditions, which include deficiencies in iron, iodine, and vitamins A, B, C, and D; recommendations for diagnosis, treatment, and prevention are also given. Such deficiencies can arise easily, even when food supplements are regularly provided, if the range of foods eaten is limited. Where rations are provided to a population that lacks ready access to other foods, including fresh foods, for more than a month, it is essential to ensure that they contain appropriate quantities of vitamin A, thiamine, riboflavin, vitamin C, iron, iodine, and folic acid.

Table 1 gives the recommended average daily per capita intakes of various specific nutrients for a typical population requiring emergency food aid in a developing country.

Monitoring the adequacy of food access and intake

Household food security is an essential element both of initial assessment (rapid assessment phase) and of emergency monitoring thereafter. Its assessment is a complex process, beyond the scope of this manual, but some procedures are outlined in another WHO publication.[2] A formal methodology is still under development.

Table 1 *Recommended mean daily per capita nutrient intakes for a typical population requiring emergency food aid in a developing country*

Nutrient	Recommended daily intake
Vitamin A (retinol) equivalents	500 μg
Vitamin D	3.8 μg
Thiamine (vitamin B_1)	0.9 mg
Riboflavin (vitamin B_2)	1.4 mg
Niacin equivalents	12.0 mg
Folic acid	160 μg
Vitamin B_{12}	0.9 μg
Vitamin C (ascorbic acid)	28 mg
Iodine	150 μg
Iron	22 mg[a]
Calcium	0.5 g

[a] From a diet that provides iron of low or very low bioavailability.

[1] *Fats and oils in human nutrition. Report of a joint FAO/WHO expert consultation*. Rome, Food and Agriculture Organization of the United Nations, 1994 (FAO Food and Nutrition Paper, No. 57).

[2] *Rapid health assessment protocols for emergencies*. Geneva, World Health Organization, 1999.

Household food security is measured in terms of household resources and access to food, including home-produced foods, foods available on the market, and wild foods, and income generated by sale of assets. Area assessments of food production potential and food availability are essential and are usually undertaken by local government or agriculture services. Market surveys identify the types and quantities of foods available on local markets — and preferably prices as well. This allows the adequacy of, and trends in, household food access to be at least partially assessed, especially if such surveys are made over a period of time.

The household food security assessment is essential to the decision on whether food distribution — either a full ration (providing all nutritional requirements) or a partial ration (supplementing whatever is available from local sources) — is needed for an at-risk or affected population.

Even if food is available in sufficient quantity and of appropriate quality to meet the daily energy, protein, and other requirements of a population in an emergency situation, there may still be problems that result in inequitable food distribution and therefore hungry or malnourished children, families, and other groups.

The methodology for measuring malnutrition is described in Chapter 3 and Annex 3. If there is no evidence of malnutrition (either protein–energy or micronutrient) in the population, it is clear that food intakes have been sufficient. However, where malnutrition is present, or when inequitable ration distribution seems to be a possibility, monitoring of adequacy of food intakes in families or vulnerable subgroups in the population becomes a vital management tool. By comparing intake of nutrients with nutrient requirements, monitoring will help to identify:

- which subgroups are receiving or consuming insufficient or excessive food and why;
- logistic difficulties in general ration distribution systems;
- vulnerable groups that may require selective targeting with supplementary rations;
- whether the nutrient content of general rations is, in fact, sufficient;
- how much food from local markets is available or being utilized;
- how much food is being utilized as a barter commodity to obtain other essentials;
- underlying causes of malnutrition.

Monitoring access to and intake of food can be approached in several different ways, but a useful and time-saving first step is to select 30 families from camp registration data where these are available. By comparing the theoretical nutrient requirements with the theoretical food provisions for each family, the proportion of families receiving too little or too much can be calculated. This is a valuable first step, before market surveys, household surveys, or food basket surveys (see Annex 7) are undertaken.

CHAPTER 2

Major nutritional deficiency diseases in emergencies

Protein–energy malnutrition (PEM) is likely to be the major health problem and a leading cause, directly or indirectly, of death during an emergency. Children under 5 years of age are usually the worst affected, but older children and adults are often also affected or at risk. The condition takes several forms:

- **Marasmus** — characterized by severe wasting of fat and muscle, which the body breaks down for energy, leaving "skin and bones". This is the most common form of PEM in nutritional emergencies.
- **Kwashiorkor** — characterized essentially by oedema (usually starting in the feet and legs); sometimes accompanied by a skin rash and/or changes in hair colour (greyish or reddish).
- **Marasmic kwashiorkor** — characterized by a combination of severe wasting and oedema.

Micronutrient deficiencies in an emergency situation are among the main causes of long-lasting or permanent disability, and most of them are associated with an increased risk of morbidity and mortality. It is useful to distinguish between the deficiencies that are common to many populations, particularly in developing countries, such as iron, iodine, and vitamin A deficiencies, and those that are more specifically seen in emergencies, such as thiamine, vitamin B, and vitamin C deficiencies, and must be looked for systematically.

- **Iron deficiency and anaemia** are most prevalent and severe in young children (aged 6–24 months) and women of reproductive age (particularly pregnant women). Anaemia develops slowly and is not clinically apparent until it becomes severe, even though there are functional consequences before this stage. In addition to anaemia, the major manifestations of iron deficiency are:
  - in children and adolescents, impairment of cognitive functions and attentiveness;
  - in pregnant women, increased risk of low-birth-weight infants, and of perinatal and maternal mortality;
  - in all individuals, reduced work capacity and impaired cognition.
- **Iodine deficiency** is a "geographical" disease, present in most countries of the developing world. It occurs in areas where the soil is poor in iodine and the iodine content of plant foods consequently low, resulting in low iodine intake in the population. Young children and pregnant women are the most vulnerable to iodine deficiency. Iodine deficiency is the main cause of preventable brain damage in childhood, and gives rise to stillbirths and miscarriages, varying degrees of mental retardation, and goitre.
- **Vitamin A deficiency** occurs in several developing countries and is the main cause of preventable blindness in childhood. In addition to night blindness and ocular lesions of varying severity, called xerophthalmia, vitamin A deficiency is associated with an increased risk of mortality, especially among children with measles. Young children and pregnant women are the most vulnerable to vitamin A deficiency.

Prevention of micronutrient deficiency aims to increase the body's stores of micronutrients so that the individual can better withstand any sudden reduction in micronutrient intake or increase in demand. In practice, this involves providing the relevant micronutrients in appropriate quantities, ideally by improving the diet and increasing the consumption of micronutrient-rich foods. Unless and until this can be done, the alternative is to provide micronutrient supplements and foods fortified with micronutrients. In most cases, the most effective strategy is to combine dietary approaches, including supplementation and food fortification.

Treatment of micronutrient deficiency involves administration of appropriate doses of the missing micronutrients in medicinal form.

Protein–energy malnutrition

Causes and consequences

Even in normal times, protein–energy malnutrition (PEM) is a problem in many developing countries, most commonly affecting children between the ages of 6 months and 5 years.

The condition may result from lack of food or from infections that cause loss of appetite while increasing the body's nutrient requirements and losses (see Chapter 6). Children between 12 and 36 months old are especially at risk since they are the most vulnerable to infections such as gastroenteritis and measles. Chronic PEM has many short-term and long-term physical and mental effects, including growth retardation, lowered resistance to infections, and increased mortality rates in young children.

In times of nutritional emergency it is primarily the more acute forms of PEM that have to be dealt with. These are characterized by a rapid loss of weight and may affect significantly larger numbers of older children, adolescents, and adults than usual.

In many emergencies, only a small proportion of the total population shows clinical signs of severe PEM, yet for each case of severe PEM there may be 10 cases of moderate PEM and many more of undernutrition. If moderate malnutrition is left untreated, it may rapidly become severe, and case-fatality rates in severe PEM (especially kwashiorkor) can be very high. The malnutrition problem may therefore be much more common and serious in the community than a small number of severe PEM cases would suggest.

Death rates are high among children with untreated PEM, and the risk of dying increases with the severity of the condition. Even after treatment is started it is not uncommon for deaths to result from electrolyte imbalance, hypoglycaemia, hypothermia, or complicating infections.

Symptoms and signs

The clinical signs and symptoms of protein–energy malnutrition are summarized in Table 2.

Table 2 *Main clinical symptoms and signs of protein–energy malnutrition*

Population group	Clinical symptom/sign	
	Always present	Sometimes present
Children:		
Marasmus	Wasting	Hunger Wizened appearance
Kwashiorkor	Oedema	Mental change: irritability Poor appetite Skin change: "flaky-paint" dermatosis Hair: sparse, loose, straight
Marasmic kwashiorkor	Wasting + oedema	Any of the above symptoms and signs
Adults	Wasting and weakness	Oedema Mental change

Fig. 1 Child suffering from nutritional marasmus

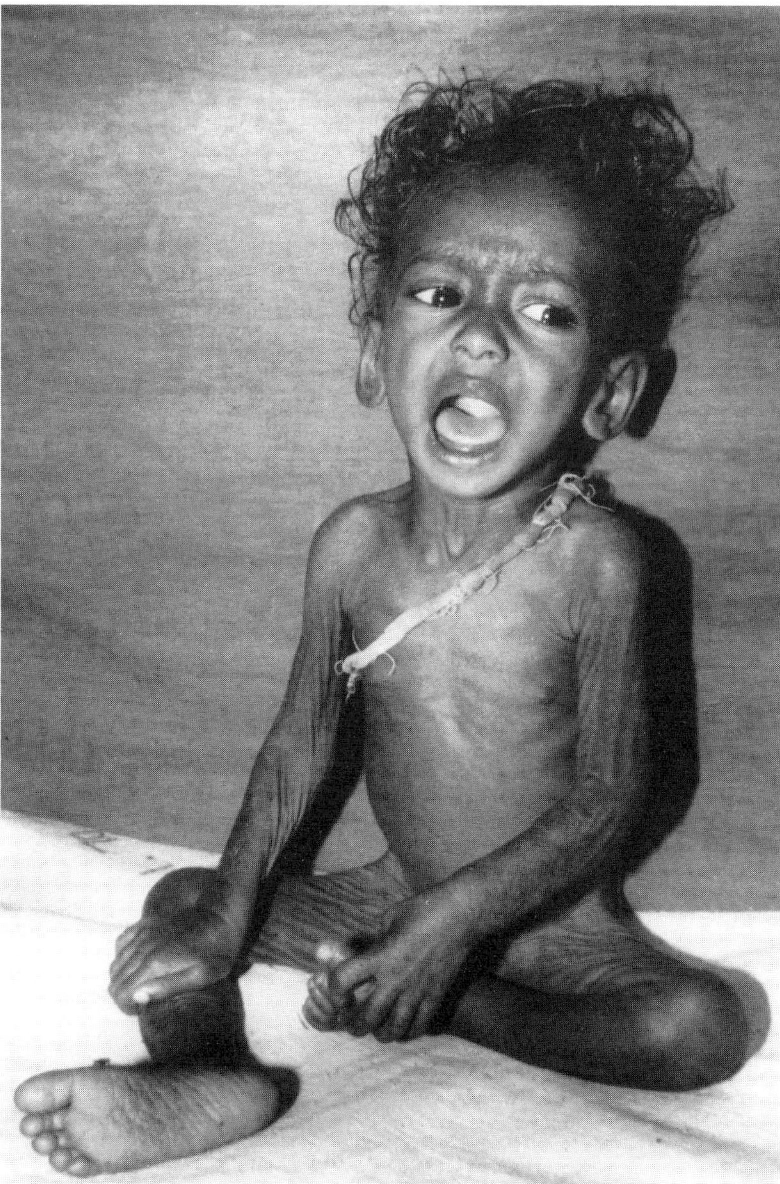

Nutritional marasmus results from prolonged starvation (see Fig. 1). Marasmus may also result from chronic or recurring infections with marginal food intake, and is then called *secondary marasmus*. The main sign is a severe wasting away of fat and muscle. The affected child (or adult) is very thin ("skin and bones"), most of the fat and muscle mass having been expended to provide energy. Marasmus is the most frequent form of PEM in conditions of severe food shortage.

Associated signs of the condition can be:

- A thin "old man" face.
- "Baggy pants" (the loose skin of the buttocks hanging down).

Fig. 2 A severe case of kwashiorkor showing oedema and skin and hair changes

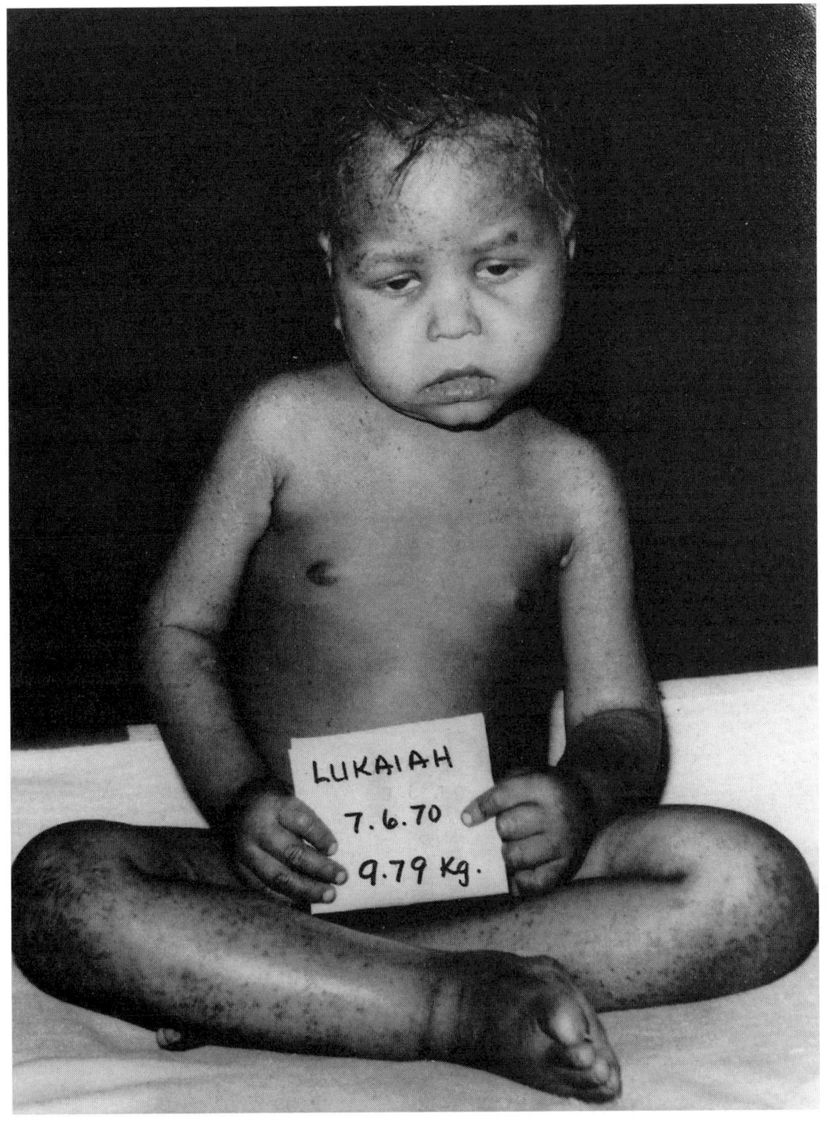

- Affected children may appear to be alert in spite of their condition.
- There is no oedema (swelling that pits on pressure) of the lower extremities.
- Ribs are very prominent.

Kwashiorkor (see Figs 2 and 3) usually affects children aged 1–4 years, although it also occurs in older children and adults. The main sign is oedema, usually starting in the legs and feet and spreading, in more advanced cases, to the hands and face. Oedema may be detected by the production of a definite pit as a result of moderate pressure for 3 seconds with the thumb over the lower end of the tibia. Because of oedema, children with kwashiorkor may look "fat" so that their parents regard them as well fed.

Associated signs can be:

Fig. 3 A 13-month-old Ugandan boy with severe kwashiorkor

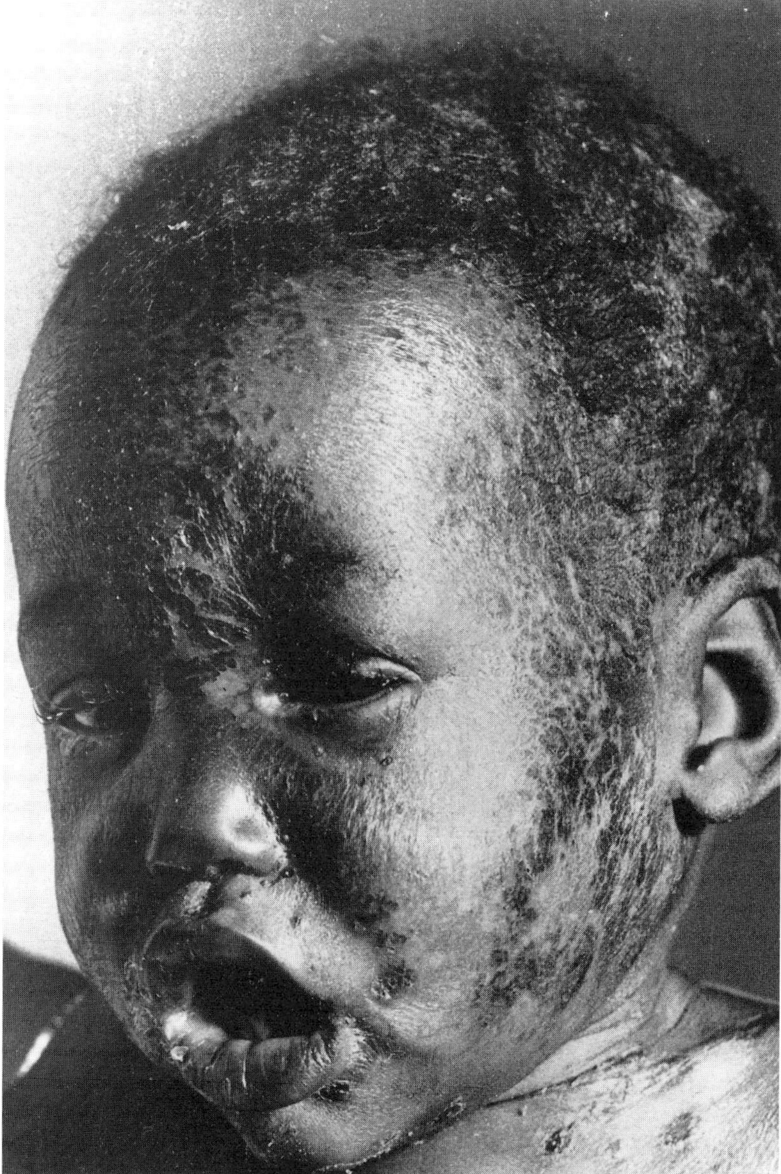

- Hair changes: loss of pigmentation; curly hair becomes straight (an African child may appear to have much longer hair than usual); easy pluckability (the hair comes out easily with a very gentle pull).
- Skin lesions and depigmentation: dark skin may become lighter in some places, especially in the skin folds; outer layers of skin may peel off (especially on the legs), and ulceration may occur; the lesions may resemble burns.
- Children with kwashiorkor are usually apathetic, miserable, and irritable. They show no signs of hunger, and it is difficult to persuade them to eat.

The associated signs of kwashiorkor do not always occur. In some cases, oedema may be the only visible sign, while in others all the signs may be present.

Marasmic kwashiorkor is a mixed form of PEM, with oedema occurring in children who are otherwise marasmic and who may or may not have other signs of kwashiorkor.

Clinical features of PEM in older children and adults are basically similar to those in young children, but skin and hair signs are less evident. The main features are wasting, or cachexia in severe cases, with or without oedema which may be generalized or mainly in dependent parts, such as feet and legs.

Treatment

Infants and children suffering from severe forms of protein–energy malnutrition must be treated as soon as possible, otherwise they are very likely to die. The treatment, which consists of three well-defined phases, is described in Chapter 5. The reader is also referred to the WHO publication *Management of severe malnutrition: a manual for physicians and other senior health workers.*[1]

Micronutrient deficiencies and nutritional relief

Micronutrient deficiencies occur all over the world but particularly in developing countries. Not all populations are equally at risk of each type of micronutrient deficiency: while iron deficiency anaemia may affect all countries, the likelihood of iodine and vitamin A deficiency varies from region to region. Special attention should therefore be given to population groups who come from areas of known specific deficiencies.

The most effective way to prevent micronutrient deficiency is to provide a diet that is diversified and includes fresh foods. For practical and logistic reasons, however, emergency food supplies usually consist of three or four basic items that are rarely changed and do not normally include fresh foods. A population that has to depend entirely on such a limited range of food items for more than 2 months runs the risk of developing nutritional deficiencies, especially scurvy (from lack of vitamin C) and pellagra (from lack of niacin).

There are several approaches to preventing onset of micronutrient deficiencies in emergency situations affecting large populations:

- Increasing the daily ration will allow a surplus to be sold for other purposes. It has been found that refugees receiving increased rations in fact consume a greater amount of fruit and vegetables;[2] however, it would clearly be advisable to provide information to the households concerned, at the same time as rations, about micronutrient deficiencies and the importance of fruits and vegetables, so as to encourage the regular purchase of those foods.
- Varying the composition of the food basket, so that it contains more micronutrient-rich foods such as pulses (e.g. dried beans), groundnuts, fresh fruits and vegetables, and red palm oil. Pulses and groundnuts are easily obtainable. Fresh fruits and vegetables can be procured locally if they are readily

---

[1] *Management of severe malnutrition: a manual for physicians and other senior health workers.* Geneva, World Health Organization, 1999.

[2] Hansch S. Diet and ration use in Central American refugee camps. *Journal of refugee studies*, 1992, 5(4): 300–312.

(or potentially) available; if not, bringing them from a substantial distance is likely to be too costly. A better alternative is local production of fruits and vegetables in home gardens — this should be encouraged wherever agricultural conditions permit.

- Including micronutrient-fortified foods in the ration, e.g. cereals or cereal/pulse blends (see Annex 5) enriched with iron and/or vitamins A and B complex, iodized salt, vitamin A-enriched dried skim milk, or vegetable oils. Fortified products are considerably more costly than non-fortified ones and there has to be a trade-off: supplying more fortified products is likely to mean that a lesser total quantity of food is available.
- Providing supplementation when there is likely to be a specific deficiency, for instance when populations come from an area at known risk of that deficiency or are fed on a diet that is poor in particular micronutrients.

If clinical signs of deficiencies are already widespread, or if evaluation of dietary intake indicates specific deficiencies, the following measures are recommended:

- improving the diet by adding foods rich in the missing micronutrient(s), e.g. fresh vegetables and whole-grain processed cereals (ideally in ground form);
- supplementation with the missing micronutrient(s) until such time as the diet provides sufficient quantities to prevent deficiencies;
- when necessary, treatment of individuals with overt signs and symptoms of acute deficiencies.

The main clinical signs and symptoms of micronutrient deficiencies are summarized in Table 3.

Iron deficiency and anaemia

Causes and consequences

Iron deficiency is the world's most widespread nutritional disorder and is more prevalent in developing countries and among poor populations. It particularly affects young children, especially low-birth-weight infants, and women of reproductive age, especially those who are pregnant: in developing countries, nearly all young children and pregnant women have low body iron stores. Iron deficiency is the main cause of anaemia and is usually associated with other factors that cause or contribute to anaemia, such as nutritional deficiencies (folic acid, vitamins A and B), malaria, intestinal parasitic infestations (especially hookworm, schistosomiasis, and amoebiasis), and chronic infections including HIV infection. This indicates the importance of assessing the extent of the contribution made by these factors when deciding on a strategy for anaemia control.

Iron is present in foods of both animal and vegetable origin, but it is absorbed better from those of animal origin. Foods relatively rich in iron include red meat (especially liver), dark green leafy vegetables, pulses (e.g. beans), and tubers. Absorption of iron can be greatly enhanced by consuming foods of animal origin and also by increasing dietary vitamin C content (doubling the vitamin C content of a normal diet will double iron absorption). The presence of certain substances in cereals and in tea and coffee seriously inhibits iron absorption. Breast

***Table 3** Main clinical symptoms and signs of nutritional deficiencies and disorders*

Deficiency/disorder	Clinical symptom/sign	
	Always present	**Sometimes present**
Iron-deficiency anaemia:		
Severe	Tiredness Pallor (palms, tongue)	Breathlessness Pallor (conjunctiva) History/signs of blood loss
Mild/moderate	No definite pallor	Tiredness History/signs of blood loss
Vitamin A deficiency (VAD):		
(X1B)	Xerosis of conjunctiva	Bitot's spots
(X2)	Xerosis of cornea	
(X3A)	Xerosis of cornea + ulcer	
(X3B)	Keratomalacia	
(XS)	Corneal scar + history of VAD	
Iodine deficiency disorders:		
Goitre	Thyroid enlargement	
Cretinism	Mental defect	Deaf-mutism Squint Spastic paralysis
Beriberi:		
Infantile	Vomiting, restlessness, pallor → breathlessness, cyanosis "Wet" form: cardiac enlargement	Cardiac failure, convulsions, facial contractions, coma, aphonia (hoarseness)
Older child/adult	"Dry" form: sensory disturbances, progressive weakness, diminished reflexes	Congestive heart failure, oedema Weight loss Difficulty in squatting; foot-drop; eventual paralysis
Pellagra	Diarrhoea Dermatosis (exposed parts) Dementia	
Scurvy:		
Infantile	Pseudoparalysis due to painful subperiosteal haemorrhages (usually arms or legs)	Frog-like contracted position
Older child/adult	Bleeding, purple, swollen gums (no pus)	Easy bruising Swollen, painful, large joints

milk has a low iron content but the iron is better absorbed than that in cow's milk. In developing countries, typical diets lack variety and may be based on cereals that are low in iron and contain substances that inhibit iron absorption. The risk of iron deficiency — and of consequent anaemia — is therefore high.

Iron deficiency gives rise to functional consequences before anaemia becomes clinically apparent. In infants and young children, these consequences include impaired psychomotor development and coordination, impaired scholastic achievement, reduced physical activity, and behavioural effects such as inattention and fatigue. In adults of both sexes, iron deficiency reduces work capacity and lowers resistance to fatigue.[1]

[1] DeMaeyer EM et al. *Preventing and controlling iron deficiency anaemia through primary health care: a guide for health administrators and programme managers.* Geneva, World Health Organization, 1989.

Table 4 *Haemoglobin levels and erythrocyte volume fraction (haematocrit) values indicative of anaemia*

Age/sex group	Haemoglobin level (g/litre)[a]	Erythrocyte volume fraction
Children, 6 months to 2 years	<110	<0.33
Children, 5–11 years	<115	<0.34
Children, 12–14 years	<120	<0.36
Adult males	<130	<0.39
Non-pregnant women	<120	<0.36
Pregnant women	<110	<0.33

[a] Values given are for a population living at sea level. To correct for altitude, add 1.0 g/litre for each 100 m above 1000 m altitude, up to 3000 m.

Table 5 *Criteria for severity of anaemia*

Severity of anaemia	Pregnant women and children under 6 years		Non-pregnant women and children 6–14 years	
	Haemoglobin (g/litre)	Erythrocyte volume fraction	Haemoglobin (g/litre)	Erythrocyte volume fraction
"Mild"[a]	100–109	0.30–0.32	110–119	0.33–0.35
Moderate	70–99	0.21–0.29	80–109	0.24–0.32
Severe	<70	<0.21	<80	<0.24

[a] "Mild" is a misnomer: iron deficiency is already advanced by the time anaemia is detected. The deficiency has functional consequences even when no anaemia is clinically apparent.

In pregnant women, anaemia resulting from iron deficiency is associated with an increased risk of maternal and fetal mortality and morbidity and of intra-uterine growth retardation.

Symptoms, signs and diagnosis

The symptoms and signs of anaemia — fatigue and shortness of breath, and pallor of the skin, oral mucosa, and eyelids — are nonspecific and are clinically detectable only when the anaemia is moderate or severe. Diagnosis of anaemia and assessment of its severity therefore requires measurement of the haemoglobin concentration of the circulating blood, or of the erythrocyte volume fraction (haematocrit). Various small manual or battery-operated haemoglobinometers are available and are suitable for use in the field. Measurement of erythrocyte volume fraction involves collection of a minute quantity of blood in a heparinized capillary tube, which can then be spun in a battery-operated microcentrifuge; this can also be done in the field.

Haemoglobin levels and values of erythrocyte volume fraction indicative of anaemia are given in Table 4. Laboratory methods for assessment of iron and other micronutrients are summarized in Annex 8.

For practical purposes, since the main affected groups are women and children, the cut-off points given in Table 5 can be used to distinguish mild, moderate, and severe anaemia, although these thresholds should not be regarded as rigid.

Table 6 *Proposed classification of public health significance of anaemia and iron deficiency in populations*

Category of public health significance	Prevalence of anaemia[a] (%)
High	≥40
Medium	20–40
Low	5.0–20

[a] Percentage of individuals below the cut-offs indicated in Table 5.

Criteria for public health significance of prevalence of iron deficiency and anaemia

In addition to the criteria for clinical severity of anaemia outlined in Table 5, there is a need for criteria for the epidemiological significance of anaemia in a population. A proposed classification of public health significance is given in Table 6; intervention should be seriously considered if prevalence exceeds 20%.

More details on indicators of iron deficiency are being prepared by WHO.[1]

Prevention

Prevention of iron deficiency should always be an integral component of measures taken during nutritional emergencies. It should be based on a combination of dietary approaches, including food fortification and supplementation .The main preventive measures are outlined in the following paragraphs.

Dietary improvement

Dietary improvement consists of increasing the amount of bio-available iron in the diet. This implies the provision of foods that are rich in iron, low in inhibitors of iron absorption, and high in substances that enhance absorption. Tea and coffee contain significant quantities of absorption-inhibitors and should therefore be drunk 2 hours before or after meals rather than with them. Consumption of even small amounts of meat or other foods of animal origin or of foods rich in vitamin C (e.g. fresh fruits and vegetables), as well as the regular consumption of foods rich in folid acid (particularly dark green leafy vegetables), will significantly improve the intake and absorption of iron.

Breast-feeding

Every effort should be made to promote the breast-feeding of infants and to encourage its continuation, even for sick children.

Iron-fortified foods

Although iron-fortified foods are not usually available, iron-fortified breast-milk substitutes may be available for infants who cannot be breast-fed — but should not be allowed to discourage or prevent mothers from breast-feeding their babies.

[1] *Iron deficiency anaemia: assessment, prevention and control.* In preparation (will be available on request from Programme of Nutrition, World Health Organization, 1211 Geneva 27, Switzerland).

Table 7 *Iron supplementation for children up to 24 months of age*

Prevalence of anaemia in children 6–24 months	Birth weight	Daily dose		Duration of supplementation
		Iron	Folic acid	
<40%	Normal	12.5 mg	50 μg	From 6 to 12 months of age
	Low	12.5 mg	50 μg	From 2 to 24 months of age
≥40%	Normal	12.5 mg	50 μg	From 6 to 24 months of age
	Low	12.5 mg	50 μg	From 2 to 24 months of age

Table 8 *Iron supplementation for pregnant women*

Prevalence of anaemia in pregnant women	Daily dose		Duration of supplementation
	Iron	Folic acid	
<40%	60 mg	400 μg	6 months in pregnancy
≥40%	60 mg	400 μg	6 months in pregnancy, continuing to 3 months postpartum

Supplementation

In areas where the diet supplies inadequate quantities of iron, and iron-fortified foods are not available, supplementation becomes necessary, especially for pregnant women and young children who are the most vulnerable groups. The following recommendations are based on INACG/WHO/UNICEF guidelines:[1]

- *Children up to 24 months of age.* Guidelines for iron supplementation of young children are summarized in Table 7. Low-birth-weight infants (birth weight <2500 g) usually have low body iron stores and, regardless of the prevalence of anaemia in the population, should always be given iron and folic acid supplements from the age of 2 months to 24 months. All other young children should be similarly supplemented from the age of 6 months, stopping at 12 months where anaemia prevalence is <40% and at 24 months where prevalence is 40% or more. Where there are no data on the anaemia prevalence among children aged 6–24 months, it should be assumed to be similar to that in pregnant women in the same population.

- *Pregnant women.* Guidelines for iron supplementation of pregnant women are summarized in Table 8. To prevent iron deficiency during pregnancy, supplementation should ideally be provided to non-pregnant women, and particularly adolescents. Most women, however, have low iron stores when pregnancy begins; iron demand is high during pregnancy and so the situation worsens. All women should therefore receive both iron and folic acid supplementation for at least 6 months from the start of pregnancy; where this duration of treatment cannot be achieved, the iron dose should be increased from 60 mg to 120 mg. Where the prevalence of anaemia exceeds 40%, supplementation should continue for 3 months postpartum.

[1] Stoltzfus RJ, Dreyfuss ML. *Guidelines for the use of iron supplements to prevent and treat iron deficiency anaemia.* Washington, DC, International Nutritional Anaemia Consultative Group, 1998.

Table 9 *Iron supplementation for other population groups*

Age groups	Daily iron dose
Children 2–5 years	20–30 mg
Children 6–11 years	30–60 mg
Adolescents and adults	60 mg

Table 10 *Treatment of severe anaemia*

Age group	Daily dose		Duration of treatment
	Iron	Folic acid	
Children <2 years	25 mg	100–400 μg	3 months
Children 2–12 years	120 mg	400 μg	3 months
Adolescent and adults, including pregnant women	600 mg	400 μg	3 months

- *Other population groups.* Where the prevalence of anaemia in the population is high, iron supplementation should be envisaged for children, adolescents, and adults; guidelines are given in Table 9. The efficacy and operational efficiency in field conditions of daily and weekly supplements for children and adolescents are currently being evaluated and compared.

Public health measures

In areas where there is malaria, hookworm, or schistosomiasis, measures should be taken to prevent these infections and to treat cases of active disease (see Chapter 6). Special attention should be paid to malaria prophylaxis and hookworm prevention in pregnant women and in children. In addition, avoidance of overcrowding, provision of safe water supplies and adequate sanitation, and promotion of safe food handling all help to reduce the risk of infection and consequently of anaemia.

Treatment of severe anaemia

The treatment schedule for severe iron deficiency anaemia is given in Table 10. The specified iron dosage and duration of treatment should be strictly observed. After completing the 3 months of therapeutic supplementation, infants and pregnant women should continue to receive preventive supplementation.

Severely malnourished children are also usually severely anaemic. However, iron supplementation should be delayed until a child regains his or her appetite and has started to gain weight, which is usually after 14 days of therapeutic feeding.

Adults may complain of side-effects of iron supplements, including gastric problems, nausea, headache, and black stools. These side-effects are minor and generally transient but they may affect compliance.

Iron may have toxic effects in young children if the age-specific dose for prevention or treatment of anaemia is exceeded. When mothers are given large quantities of iron for supplementation, they should be warned to keep the tablets out of the reach of children.

Iodine deficiency

Causes and consequences

Iodine deficiency occurs worldwide and is a public health problem in 130 countries. Young children and pregnant women are more susceptible to iodine deficiency than other population groups. The term "iodine-deficiency disorders" covers a wide range of adverse effects of deficiency, including thyroid enlargement (goitre) without clinical significance, miscarriages and stillbirths, neonatal and juvenile thyroid insufficiency, dwarfism, mental defects, deaf-mutism, spastic weakness, and paralysis, as well as lesser impairments of physical and mental functions. Iodine deficiency is also the commonest preventable cause of brain damage in childhood.

Deficiency arises when dietary iodine intake does not meet requirements. The diet is likely to be deficient in iodine wherever the soil content of iodine is low, which is often the case in mountainous regions. In addition, certain foods contain goitrogens — substances that inhibit iodine absorption or utilization — and need to be detoxified before being consumed.

Emergencies *per se* do not normally provoke iodine-deficiency disorders, but displaced populations may be relocated to iodine-deficient areas. In such cases it becomes important to provide iodine in order to prevent the consequences of deficiency.

Diagnosis and assessment

It is essential to assess the extent and severity of iodine-deficiency disorders in order to determine whether there is a public health problem and whether or not an intervention is needed. The two principal indicators are the total goitre rate and urinary iodine levels (see Table 11), both of which are normally assessed in a population of preschool children.

Prevention

Foods supplied for emergency relief, especially cereals, should normally contain enough iodine, but may have been grown in iodine-deficient soils. Only seafoods

Table 11 *Criteria for assessment of the severity of iodine-deficiency disorders*[a]

Prevalence of iodine-deficiency disorders	Indicators	
	Total goitre rate (%)	Median urinary iodine level (μg/litre)
Normal	<5.0	≥100
Mild	5.0–19.9	50–99
Moderate	20.0–29.9	20–49
Severe	≥30.0	<20

[a] Source: *Indicators for assessing iodine deficiency disorders and their control through salt iodization.* Geneva, World Health Organization, 1994 (unpublished document WHO/NUT/94.6, available on request from Programme of Nutrition, World Health Organization, 1211 Geneva 27, Switzerland).

Table 12 *Doses and duration of effect of iodized oil*[a]

Age groups	Oral doses (mg) for effects lasting:			Intramuscular dose (ml) for effect lasting >1 year
	3 months	6 months	12 months	
Infants <1 year	20–40	50–100	100–300	0.5
Children 1–5 years	40–100	100–300	300–480	1.0
Children 5–16 years	100–200	200–480	400–960	1.0
Non-pregnant women of childbearing age	100–200	200–480	400–960	1.0
Pregnant women	50–100	100–300	300–480	1.0
Males 16–45 years	100–200	200–480	400–960	1.0

[a] Commercially available capsules of iodized oil for oral administration commonly contain about 200 mg iodine; an appropriate preparation for intramuscular injection contains about 480 mg of iodine/ml.

are relatively rich in iodine, containing about 100 μg per 100 g. The daily adult iodine requirement is approximately 150 μg, rising to 200 μg during pregnancy. Emergency rations designed for general distribution may supply about 50 g of fish per day but this would not provide enough iodine to meet the daily requirement fully.

Prevention of iodine deficiency is usually achieved through the use of iodized salt. This is available in most countries where iodine-deficiency disorders are prevalent, but not all. In undertaking either general or selective feeding programmes (see Chapters 4 and 5, respectively), it is important to ascertain whether iodized salt is available in the area. To meet iodine requirements — that is, 150 μg/day — via iodized salt, and assuming that the daily per capita salt consumption is 10 g,[1] the iodine concentration in salt should be in the range 20–40 mg iodine (or 34–66 mg of potassium iodate) per kg.

In some areas, particularly the most remote, iodized salt may not be available. An alternative solution is to provide iodized oil, administered either orally every 3, 6, or 12 months or by intramuscular injection every 2 years. Clearly, oral administration will be successful only if potential recipients can be contacted at least once a year; otherwise 2-yearly intramuscular injections are to be preferred. Doses and duration of effects are summarized in Table 12.

Vitamin A deficiency, including xerophthalmia

Causes and consequences

Vitamin A deficiency is the world's leading cause of preventable blindness in young children and contributes significantly to the high death rates of infants and young children in malnourished communities. The condition is common among displaced populations. Vitamin A supplementation of children living in areas deficient in the vitamin increases their chances of survival: risk of mortality from measles is reduced by about 50% and overall mortality by 25–35%.

[1] *Recommended iodine levels in salt and guidelines for monitoring their adequacy and effectiveness.* Geneva, World Health Organization, 1996 (unpublished document WHO/NUT/96.13, available on request from Programme of Nutrition, World Health Organization, 1211 Geneva 27, Switzerland).

In poor communities most dietary vitamin A is derived from green and yellow vegetables and fruits, including dark green leafy vegetables (e.g. amaranth), carrots, pumpkins, mangoes, and papayas; red palm oil is a particularly rich source. Vitamin A is stored in the liver. In marginally malnourished children, however, these stores are not large enough to withstand a sudden deterioration in the diet or to meet the increased demand for vitamin A that arises with diarrhoea or infection.

Since fruits and vegetables are only available seasonally in many countries, a higher incidence of vitamin A deficiency may occur towards the end of the dry season when such produce is scarce and liver stores of the vitamin may be depleted.

Symptoms and signs

Vitamin A deficiency is a systemic disease that affects cells and organs throughout the body, with epithelial changes in the respiratory, urinary, and intestinal tracts occurring relatively early. Only the ocular changes, however, are readily visible and it is for this reason that they are used for diagnosis of the deficiency. As vitamin A stores are progressively depleted, the ocular changes — or xerophthalmia — become more severe.

Night blindness is the first ocular manifestation of vitamin A deficiency and the most prevalent. In a preschool child it is a good indication of vitamin A deficiency. The child is unable to see clearly in dim light, such as inside a hut or after sundown, when normal individuals can still see reasonably well. It can be difficult to confirm loss of dim-light vision in small children. However, there may be a local dialect word for the condition, often indicating that the child easily bumps into objects after dusk; if this term is used, mothers who are questioned may be able to recognize that their children's dim-light vision is impaired.

Xerophthalmia is the term given to the eye symptoms and signs resulting from vitamin A deficiency (see Fig. 4). Table 13 lists the various lesions of the disorder. Xerophthalmia is associated with high mortality rates.

Prevention

During a famine, the population becomes malnourished and body reserves of vitamin A are severely depleted, so that individuals are particularly susceptible to vitamin A deficiency. Measures for preventing vitamin A deficiency should be initiated as a priority procedure if *any one* of the following criteria is met:

- The population originates from an area that is known or presumed to be deficient in vitamin A.
- Active xerophthalmia (night blindness, Bitot's spots, corneal xerosis, or keratomalacia) is present in the population.
- The population has been deprived of its normal food supply for several months and is subsisting on relief rations that are not fortified with vitamin A.
- Protein–energy malnutrition and/or diarrhoeal diseases are prevalent, or measles occurs in epidemic proportions.

Fig. 4 ***Xerophthalmia is difficult to detect and children are often brought to hospital too late to save their eyesight***

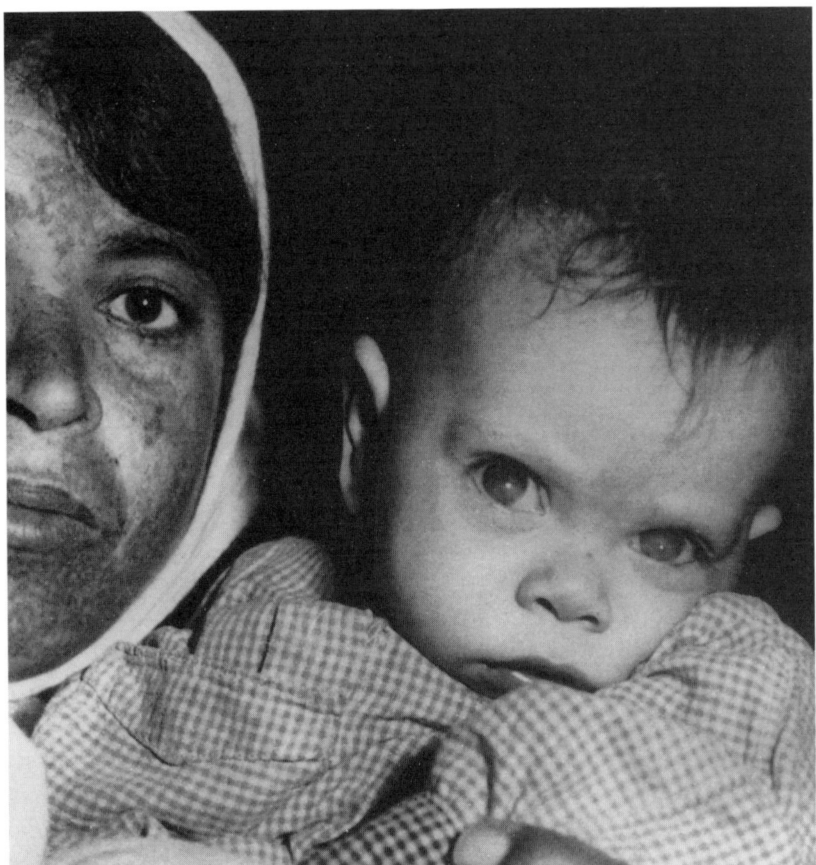

Table 13 *Classification of xerophthalmia*

Classification	Lesions of xerophthalmia	Prognosis
XN	Night blindness	These conditions are reversible and usually respond to vitamin A therapy
X1A	Conjunctival xerosis	
X1B	Bitot's spot. Dryness and apparent roughness of the conjunctiva, often accompanied by foamy or cheesy patches near the outer edge of the iris, which are called Bitot's spot.	
X2	Corneal xerosis, characterized by dryness, dullness, or clouding (milky appearance) of the cornea.	
X3A, X3B	Corneal ulceration/keratomalacia: softening and ulceration of the cornea that is the most severe stage of xerophthalmia. It is sometimes followed by perforation of the cornea, which leads to the loss of eye contents and permanent blindness. Ulceration and perforation may occur alarmingly fast (within a matter of hours), especially in young children who have measles or some other acute febrile illness.	These stages are not reversible and leave sequelae
XS	Corneal scars	
SF	Xerophthalmic fundus	

Prevention and control of vitamin A deficiency should always be an integral part of relief operations during famine. The main preventive measures are the following:

- measles immunization;
- high-dose vitamin A supplements;
- encouragement of breast-feeding, which should be continued during illnesses, including diarrhoea;
- promotion of local production, marketing, and consumption of green leafy vegetables and yellow vegetables and fruits, and consumption of animal products rich in vitamin A;
- relief foods fortified with vitamin A, particularly those destined for vulnerable groups;
- environmental sanitation and personal hygiene measures, especially those designed to prevent diarrhoeal disease.

Most dried skim milk, some vegetable oil, and various cereal blends are fortified with vitamin A. However, if foods are not labelled as fortified, it should be assumed that they are not and they should not be relied upon as a supplementary dietary source of vitamin A. Because the vitamin A content of relief foods is often unknown, periodic mass distribution of high-dose vitamin A supplements may be required.

Wherever possible, the production of green leafy vegetables and red/yellow fruits and vegetables in family and community gardens should be promoted during relief and rehabilitation efforts. Consumption of these foods, especially by infants during the complementary feeding period (from 6 months onwards), young children, and pregnant or lactating women, should be encouraged.

Infants and preschool-age children, as well as pregnant and lactating women, should have priority access to supplementary relief foods containing natural vitamin A or fortified with vitamin A.

Table 14 shows the schedules for the prophylactic use of vitamin A supplements in emergency relief operations. They apply primarily to famine conditions in which a population is malnourished and likely to have minimal liver stores of vitamin A, especially when it meets any of the criteria on page 24.

Table 14 *Vitamin A deficiency prevention schedule in emergencies*

Population group	Oral vitamin A dosage
Infants <6 months of age whose mothers have received no vitamin A supplement or who are not breast-fed	50 000 IU, once
Infants 6–12 months of age	100 000 IU, every 4–6 months
Children >1 year of age	200 000 IU, every 4–6 months[a]
Pregnant and other fertile women	Not more than 10 000 IU daily
Lactating women	200 000 IU once during first 8 weeks after delivery[b]

[a] Adequate protection can also be achieved with smaller, more frequent doses, e.g. 10 000 IU weekly or 50 000 IU monthly.

[b] If the mother is not lactating, the supplement should be given within 6 weeks of delivery to prevent any risk of teratogenicity in a subsequent pregnancy.

Treatment

Xerophthalmia is a medical emergency that must be promptly treated.

Children and adult males

The recommended schedule for treatment of xerophthalmia in children and adult males is shown in Table 15.

Women of reproductive age

Women of reproductive age with night blindness or Bitot's spots should receive daily vitamin A doses not exceeding 10 000 IU or weekly doses not exceeding 25 000 IU. All women of childbearing age — whether or not they are pregnant — who exhibit severe signs of active xerophthalmia (i.e. acute corneal lesions) should be treated with a daily vitamin A dose of 5000–10 000 IU or a weekly dose of 25 000 IU for at least 4 weeks.

Pregnant women

Pregnant women are at increased risk of vitamin A deficiency, particularly in areas that are deficient in the vitamin, and may develop night blindness, especially during the third trimester. To improve the vitamin A status of both mother and fetus, the mother should consume a diet containing adequate amounts of vitamin A and/or should receive frequent small doses of vitamin A not exceeding 10 000 IU daily or 25 000 IU weekly.

When there are severe signs of active xerophthalmia, it becomes essential to weigh the possible teratogenic and other effects on the fetus of a high vitamin A dose against the possible serious consequences for both mother and fetus of vitamin A deficiency. In these circumstances, the high-dose treatment schedule given in Table 15 may be followed.

High-risk groups

Infants and children with severe protein–energy malnutrition — as well as measles, diarrhoea, respiratory diseases, chickenpox, and other serious infections — are at increased risk of vitamin A deficiency, as are children living in the same house or community as others with xerophthalmia. Vitamin A supplementation of such children helps to restore body reserves of the vitamin, protect again deficiency, and limit the severity of subsequent infections. The prevention schedule for high-risk children is given in Table 16. If a child has received a routine dose

Table 15 *Vitamin A dosage schedule for treatment of xerophthalmia*

Timing	Oral vitamin A dosage[a]
Immediately on diagnosis:	
<6 months of age	50 000 IU
6–12 months of age	100 000 IU
>1 year of age	200 000 IU
Following day	Same age-specific dose
At least 2 weeks later	Same age-specific dose

[a] Preferably as an oil-based preparation.

Table 16 *Vitamin A deficiency prevention schedule for high-risk children*

Age groups	Vitamin A dosage
Infants <6 months of age	50 000 IU
Infants 6–12 months of age	100 000 IU
Children >1 year of age	200 000 IU

of vitamin A within the previous 30 days, no additional dose should be given. In areas where measles is especially severe and vitamin A deficiency endemic, the full vitamin A treatment indicated in Table 15 should be given.

Supply of vitamin A

Currently the most appropriate vitamin A preparation is the soft gelatin capsule, which contains 200 000 IU of vitamin A and 40 IU of vitamin E. Vitamin A capsules can be obtained through UNICEF and should be included in any relief agency's list of essential drugs. They have a shelf-life of up to 2 years when stored under suitable conditions. To provide a half dose of vitamin A, i.e. 100 000 IU, the nipple of a capsule should be cut with scissors and 2–3 drops squeezed out; the remaining liquid can then be squeezed into a child's mouth. Sugar-coated tablets containing 10 000 IU of vitamin A should be used if daily distribution to pregnant and other fertile women is planned. Capsules and tablets should be stored centrally for periodic mass distribution but should also be made available to hospitals and feeding centres. Preventive doses should be distributed to people when they are first seen and, if at all possible, records should be kept to avoid under- or over-dosing.

Side-effects of high doses of vitamin A — chiefly bulging fontanelle, nausea, vomiting, and somnolence — occur in a small percentage of young children, especially infants. However, the side-effects are transient and disappear within hours.

Vitamin C deficiency (scurvy)

Causes and consequences

Vitamin C (ascorbic acid) is found mainly in fresh fruits (especially citrus fruits) and vegetables, including green leafy vegetables. It is also present in quite substantial quantities in tubers such as potatoes and sweet potatoes and is found in sprouted pulses. At least half of the vitamin content is destroyed by cooking except for very short periods — and losses are greater if the cooking water is thrown away. Because famine often occurs in arid areas and in times of drought, fresh fruits and vegetables are frequently in short supply and are expensive if they have to be bought. For all these reasons scurvy is still unacceptably common among poor populations affected by drought or famine. Prevalence is generally higher among pregnant and lactating women and adolescent males.

Apart from being essential to prevent scurvy, vitamin C also greatly favours the absorption of iron: doubling vitamin C intake approximately doubles the amount of iron absorbed from a mainly vegetable diet.

Table 17 *Options for the prevention of vitamin C deficiency in an emergency*

A. Local production of fruits/vegetables easy

Fruits/vegetables immediately available:

1. Add some fruits/vegetables to the ration
2. Encourage barter or purchase by providing 10% extra ration

Fruits/vegetables not immediately available:

3. Encourage household food production by providing necessary inputs

B. Local production of fruits/vegetables not easy

Provision of commodities fortified with vitamin C:

4. Fortified cereal flour or fortified sugar
5. Fortified cereal/pulse blended food (120 mg vitamin C per ration)
6. Other vitamin C-rich foods, e.g. fortified tomato paste, orange juice powder

Provision of vitamin C supplements:

7. Distribution of vitamin C tablets at least weekly

Breast milk is a good source of vitamin C. Infants who are not breast-fed are particularly prone to scurvy, and it is usually necessary to provide them with fruit juice or some other source of the vitamin. Fresh milk of animals including cows, camels, and goats contains good amounts of vitamin C. However, in poor countries such milk usually has to be boiled to minimize the risk of infection; this tends to destroy the vitamin C and so the risk of scurvy persists.

Symptoms and signs

The symptoms and signs of scurvy include bleeding and swollen gums, particularly between the teeth, and swollen, painful joints, especially knees, hips, and elbows. Bleeding may take place in any tissue, however, resulting in easy bruising and even anaemia. Bleeding and swollen gums can also be caused by gingivitis, but this disorder may be distinguished by the presence of pus and absence of hypertrophy.

Haemorrhages on the surface of bone (subperiosteal haemorrhages) are painful and can cause pseudoparalysis. Infants are particularly susceptible and often assume "frog-like" contracted positions. Adults may adopt a reclining position with legs contracted and be very reluctant to stretch their legs for fear of acute pain.

Prevention

Scurvy can be prevented by the consumption of at least 10 mg of vitamin C daily in the diet. That is roughly equivalent to 15 ml of fresh citrus juice, one-quarter of an orange, a small tomato, 20 g of green leafy vegetables, or 30 g of sprouted pulses. See Table 17 for options.

Treatment

Scurvy is treated by administering 1 g of ascorbic acid daily for 2–3 weeks. Although smaller doses for shorter periods may relieve immediate symptoms and signs, the larger doses and more prolonged treatment are recommended to prevent relapse.

Vitamin B_1 deficiency (beriberi)

Causes and consequences

Deficiency of vitamin B_1 (thiamine) — beriberi — tends to be confined to areas in which polished white rice or cassava is the sole staple. It occurs especially when energy expenditure is high, e.g. in pregnant or lactating women or active young men, and energy requirements are met mainly from foods rich in carbohydrates and relatively low in thiamine.

Vitamin B_1 occurs in whole-grain cereals, especially rice, but a large part is removed in the milling process. It is therefore essential to provide whole-grain cereals, cereal flour that is only lightly milled ("high extraction" flour), or flour enriched with thiamine. If whole-grain cereals are provided, the availability and suitability of existing milling facilities should be ascertained. Facilities should be provided if there are none, and *light* milling should be recommended.

Pulses (e.g. dried beans) and groundnuts are also rich in vitamin B_1, and some vegetables are good sources. Meat and dairy products, if available, are moderately good sources.

The vitamin is highly soluble, and about half is commonly lost during the cooking of cereals and vegetables. Losses are greater if the cooking water is discarded.

Symptoms and signs

Beriberi occurs in both infants and adults, with both acute and chronic manifestations. The "wet" (acute cardiac) form may cause heart enlargement and failure leading to acute swelling (oedema), increasing breathlessness, and sudden death. In the "dry" (more chronic) form, symptoms include weakness, weight loss, and disturbance of sensation, followed by a progressive ascending paralysis of the toes, fingers, and limbs, with reduced reflexes in the limbs. If an individual cannot stand up from a squatting position without support, this may imply early beriberi (although the problem might also be PEM or anaemia).

Infantile beriberi is more often the acute cardiac form and is seen in breast-fed infants between the second and fifth months of life. Although the mother should also be checked for beriberi, she may have no clinical signs, but will have a history of a poor diet. Infantile beriberi is frequently triggered by an infection. It begins with loss of appetite, vomiting, restlessness, and pallor. Quite suddenly the infant becomes breathless and cyanotic (blue), with a weak and rapid pulse. In severe cases, aphonia is a characteristic sign — the infant appears to be crying, but little or no sound is heard. Sometimes abdominal pain, convulsions, and coma set in, and death may occur within 24–28 hours.

In older infants (7–9 months), beriberi may produce central nervous system signs, including spasmodic contraction of facial muscles and convulsions, as well as fever.

Prevention

About 1 mg of thiamine daily is sufficient to prevent beriberi. Adequate quantities can be obtained from whole-grain cereals, pulses, nuts, and red meats. When the staple cereal is polished rice or cassava, it is important to include pulses and/or nuts in the ration to avoid the risk of beriberi.

Treatment

If severe heart failure, convulsions, or coma occur in infantile beriberi, 25–50 mg of thiamine should be given very slowly intravenously, followed by a daily intramuscular dose of 10 mg for about 1 week. This should be followed by 3–5 mg of thiamine per day orally for at least 6 weeks. For less severe cases, 10 mg of thiamine per day should be given orally (or intramuscularly) during the first week, followed by 3–5 mg per day orally for at least 6 weeks.

Critically ill adults should be given 50–100 mg of thiamine very slowly intravenously, followed by the same oral doses as for infants.

Lactating women with signs of latent or mild beriberi should receive 10 mg of thiamine per day orally for 1 week, followed by 3–5 mg per day orally for at least 6 weeks to prevent the development of acute beriberi in their infants.

Niacin deficiency (pellagra)

Causes and consequences

Pellagra arises when the diet is chronically deficient in niacin (nicotinic acid) or contains excess isoleucine. This occurs mainly among populations whose staples are maize and sorghum (especially if these have been in storage for a long time) and who have little other food.

Symptoms and signs

Pellagra can be recognized by a characteristic symmetrical rash where skin is exposed to sunlight. It often causes severe diarrhoea and mental deterioration. The effects are known as "the four Ds": diarrhoea, dermatitis, dementia, and — ultimately — death. The mouth becomes sore and the tongue brilliant red or beef-red in colour, swollen, painful, and denuded. Pellagra is commonly a disease of adults, usually occurring between the ages of 20 and 50 years. It can also affect schoolchildren and adolescents, but rarely affects infants and young children.

Prevention

An average niacin intake of 15–20 mg per person per day prevents pellagra in all age groups. Food sources of niacin and niacin equivalents are pulses, nuts, lightly milled cereals, meat (especially liver), fish, milk, and cheese.

Treatment

The effect of niacin is dramatic in curing pellagra. The daily oral dosage is 300 mg, and treatment should continue for 3–4 weeks. Acute inflammation of the tongue, as well as diarrhoea, subsides in a few days and the mental symptoms usually disappear quickly. In chronic pellagra a longer recovery period is required, but appetite and general health improve rapidly. Niacin is readily absorbed from the stomach, even in individuals with severe digestive disorders, and intravenous or intramuscular administration is unnecessary. Nicotinamide is preferred for treatment since large doses of niacin cause flushing of the skin, nausea, vomiting, and tingling and numbness of the tongue and lower jaw.

Vitamin D deficiency (rickets)

Causes and consequences

Rickets is characterized by deformed, soft bones since lack of vitamin D affects the growth of bone and cartilage. Vitamin D activity is generated in the skin by the action of the ultraviolet component of sunlight. With normal, and even quite short but regular, exposure to sunlight rickets does not occur. However, if exposure to sunlight is limited by keeping infants or children indoors or because of constantly cloudy conditions, there is a risk of rickets. The condition is still very widespread in northern Africa and in southern Asian countries, and preventive measures should be routinely introduced in these areas.

Symptoms and signs

An early sign of rickets is the enlargement of bone/cartilage junctions at the ends of long bones (wrists and ankles) and in the ribs (rachitic beads). The skull develops an irregular square form with bossing, while the long bones are bowed and the pelvis deformed. Walking is delayed. Young children are more prone to recurrent respiratory infections.

Prevention

The best way to prevent rickets is by exposing the unclothed child to sunlight for 10–15 minutes daily, and/or by fortification of baby foods with vitamin D.

Treatment

Treatment consists of the oral administration of 5000 IU of vitamin D daily for 4–6 weeks, followed by 1000 IU daily for 6 months. These supplements are usually given in capsules and are commonly derived from fish liver oils.

CHAPTER 3

Assessment and surveillance of nutritional status

During a nutritional emergency, relief foods may be scarce and may need to be provided preferentially ("targeted") to the people in greatest need. Food relief programmes should be planned and implemented on the basis of an initial, rapid nutritional assessment followed by systematic surveys and continuous monitoring ("surveillance") of nutritional conditions. Individuals are selected for particular interventions by a screening process.

Suitable arrangements must be made for rapidly and objectively measuring the nutritional status of:

- **Communities** — to assess the extent and severity of malnutrition, including vitamin and mineral deficiencies; to decide whether and what type of feeding programmes are needed and to set food distribution priorities; to define the composition of emergency rations; to ensure that fuel and cooking utensils are available; and to monitor changes in nutritional status over time.
- **Individuals** — to screen (i.e. select) for supplementary or therapeutic feeding and to monitor their nutritional progress.

Children under 5 years of age are particularly susceptible to malnutrition and must be a priority target group for nutritional assistance in any food emergency. Their nutritional status is a good indicator of the overall nutritional situation in most societies, and surveys are usually based on determining the status of children aged 6–59 months (or of children 60–100 cm tall when ages are not known). However, it is also useful to survey at least some groups of adolescents and adult women and men.

Various indicators may be used to assess nutritional status:

- **Weight-for-height** measurements are the best for assessing and monitoring community nutritional status in food emergencies and for screening individuals for special nutritional assistance.
- **Body mass index**, i.e. (weight in kg)/(height in metres)^2, is used for assessing the status of adults.
- **Mid-upper arm circumference** can be used as an alternative method of initial screening.
- **Oedema** is an essential indicator when kwashiorkor is prevalent.

Weight-for-age and *height-for-age* are less useful for assessment or screening in emergencies, although they can be used for continuous monitoring of the growth velocity of individual children and in assessing long-term nutritional well-being once acute malnutrition has been dealt with.

Survey results are relevant and useful only if sampling procedures are standardized and properly applied to ensure that the individuals measured are representative of the whole population and that the results are comparable over time. Results must always be interpreted with caution, taking account of other relevant information.

Reasons for measuring malnutrition in emergencies

During a nutritional emergency, not all groups of people are equally affected; different groups therefore have different needs. Relief foods and other resources may be scarce and should be targeted as rationally as possible to the people in greatest need. Determination of nutritional status, or the level of malnutrition, is essential in three contexts:

- *Initial rapid assessment.* A rapid nutritional assessment provides a basis for planning a food relief programme and must be designed to determine the nutritional status of the population; identify the nature of any specific nutritional problems; and identify the most affected groups. The assessment should also provide the following information: an estimate of the total number of people affected and of the numbers in particular vulnerable groups; general health and environmental conditions; public health risks; immunization status; dietary habits; and the local availability of foods, fuel, and cooking utensils.
- *Individual screening.* Screening identifies individuals who need special assistance, in this case malnourished individuals eligible for special food relief (usually for themselves but sometimes for their families).
- *Nutritional surveillance of populations.* Surveillance is the process of monitoring changes over time in the nutritional status of the affected population and of different groups within the population. Combined with other information it provides a basis for adjusting food distribution priorities, and for continuing, modifying, or discontinuing particular forms of assistance.[1]

Nutritional surveys are essential tools for both initial assessments and surveillance. The purpose of this type of survey in an emergency is to assess nutritional status and to determine whether food assistance should begin, continue, or be modified. Surveys should identify differences between various population groups, villages, and camps. By periodically repeating surveys, changes over time within specific groups or communities can be monitored. A survey is not intended to monitor the progress of individual children, and it must be carried out using strict sampling procedures.

Indicators of malnutrition

Malnourished individuals may be abnormally thin and underweight for their height ("wasted") and/or abnormally short in stature with linear growth retardation ("stunted"). Body measurements provide a good indication of these different forms of malnutrition in the individual; other, community-level, indicators include clinical observations and mortality and morbidity data.

Body measurement indicators

Assessments of nutritional status in emergencies are based on body measurements, or anthropometry, particularly weight, height or length, and arm circumference (see Annex 3). These measurements are complemented by data on rates

[1] Nutritional surveillance should not be confused with the "surveillance" or follow-up of an individual child in a feeding centre or health clinic.

of oedema and by clinical observations and records. It should be noted, however, that body measurements are used as indicators of malnutrition, not of food shortage as such. Malnutrition can also be caused by infections, ignorance, or faulty feeding habits even when there is sufficient food.

Children under 5 years of age

It is inappropriate to lay down firm rules on whether surveys and intervention should be limited to children under 3 years of age or children under 5 years. In some countries, malnutrition affects almost exclusively those under 3 years; in others, children aged 3–4 years are also frequently affected. In emergency conditions the age distribution may not be the same as in "normal" times, and it is therefore desirable to include all children under 5 in at least a first, or pilot, survey. If the prevalence of malnutrition is very low among children aged 3–4 years, this group can be omitted, but in most cases its inclusion is advisable.

In normal circumstances it is also common for infants up to 6 months, or even 1 year, to be less malnourished — by anthropometric criteria — than older children (up to 35 months), and it has become traditional to limit surveys to children over 6 months (interpretation of anthropometric findings in babies also tends to be inaccurate). However, breast-milk production may be severely limited in emergency conditions (for instance, because of extreme maternal malnutrition, malaria, tuberculosis, HIV, and other chronic or recurrent infections) and infections are likely to be common in infants, even those under 6 months of age. It is therefore unwise, at least initially, to exclude infants age 0–5 months from examination.

For these reasons, reference to the "vulnerable" preschool age group in the following pages includes all children under 5 years of age. In particular circumstances, however, and if justified by pilot surveys, infants under 6 months and/or children aged 3–4 years may be discounted from this vulnerable group. A full ration is issued for each infant under 6 months and, if a mother consumes at least one-quarter of that ration daily, her additional needs for lactation will be met. Nevertheless, screening should still be carried out so that severely wasted infants are detected and can be appropriately treated.

Weight for height

Weight-for-height measurement gives a reasonably accurate estimate of body wasting and is the preferred index of nutritional status in emergencies for several reasons:

- Body weight is sensitive to rapid changes in food supply (as muscle and fat are lost), while height remains relatively constant, changing only slowly if at all.
- In children under 5 years of age, the relationship of weight to height is nearly constant, regardless of sex or race, and follows a constant evolution as age increases.
- Weight-for-height is relatively independent of a child's age, which is often difficult to ascertain reliably.

- There are good internationally accepted and globally applicable reference values of weight-for-height for this age group.
- Good software for data analysis is easily available.

The weight of an individual child is compared with that of a "reference" (well nourished) child of the same height, using tables of reference values (WHO/NCHS standards; see Annex 3). Results can be expressed in the following terms: as percentages of the reference value (e.g. 80% of median reference weight-for-height); as Z-scores or standard deviation (SD) scores, where Z-score is defined as

$$\frac{[(\text{observed value}) - (\text{median reference value})]}{\text{SD of reference population}}$$

or in relation to (i.e. above or below) certain preselected cut-off values.

The standard deviation is a measure of the spread of values in a population above and below the mean values, when these values are normally distributed. Two-thirds of the population are included in the range: mean ± 1 standard deviation. In anthropometry, the median value is generally used in preference to the mean; the median is the point with 50% of the values above it and 50% below.

It should be noted that "weight-for-height" is used here as a generic term meaning weight-for-height *or* weight-for-length. Children under 2 years of age, less than 85 cm tall, or too ill to stand should have their length measured while they are lying down. Children who are 2 years old or more, at least 85 cm tall, and able to stand should have their height measured. For children who are not stunted, height can be either measured directly or derived by subtracting 0.5 cm from length measurements (which are usually 0.5 cm greater than height values, depending on measuring techniques).

In population surveys, the following cut-off points are commonly used, and the percentage of people below the selected cut-off point is then taken as the indicator of malnutrition in the population:

- 2 SD below median of the reference population (i.e. median value minus 2 SD)
- 80% of median value for weight-for-height of the reference population
- third percentile of the reference population.

Classification according to standard deviations is recommended by WHO as the method that provides the most statistically valid measure of risk and prevalence of malnutrition. In the field it is not necessary to calculate individual Z-scores; children may be classified as above −2 SD (considered "normal"), between −2 and −3 SD (moderately wasted), or below −3 SD (severely wasted). The values for −2 SD and −3 SD are read from tables such as those in Annex 3. The Z-scores of individuals for the measurement under consideration and mean Z-scores for a population can be calculated; computer software is available for this purpose (e.g. EpiInfo[1]), or a calculator can be used.

[1] A list of distributors can be obtained from Expanded Programme on Immunization, World Health Organization, 1211 Geneva 27, Switzerland.

Table 18 *Examples of weight-for-height cut-off points for classifying individual malnourished children*

Nutritional status	Cut-off points	
	Standard deviations (SD) below reference median weight-for-height	**% of reference weight-for-height**
Three nutritional groups:		
Well nourished and mild PEM	Equal to or above −2SD	80% or above
Moderate PEM	Below −2SD, equal to or above −3SD	70–79%
Severe PEM	Below −3SD	Below 70%
Two nutritional groups:		
Well nourished and mild PEM	Equal to or above −2SD	80% or above
Moderate and severe PEM	Below −2SD	Below 80%

Percentage of the median is sometimes used, since it is simpler to calculate than Z-score or percentile. Again it is unnecessary to calculate percentage of median for each child; it is enough to classify the child in a range, e.g. <60%, 60–69%, 70–79%, ≥80%. This can be done by reference to an appropriate table.

Percentiles are useful in that they are easy to interpret. The third percentile is the level below which 3% of individuals are found in a normal, well nourished population.

Some additional cut-off points, defining other levels of severity of malnutrition, are shown in Table 18. WHO recommends the cut-offs at −2 and −3SD, or the mean Z-score. (For interpretation of the proportions below the cut-off, see pages 50–51, "Analysis, interpretation, and reporting of survey results".) The results for an under-5 child population can also be expressed as the mean Z-score, calculated from the individual weight-for-height Z-scores of each child. This mean Z-score has its own standard deviation, standard error of the mean, and coefficient of variation. Two different population Z-scores can thus be readily compared statistically to determine whether they are significantly different.

When weight-for-height surveys are performed, children with oedema should be excluded from the analysis and their number reported separately; they are considered to be severely malnourished.

Weight-for-age

Weight-for-age is not a particularly useful index for screening or for assessment surveys in nutritional emergencies. Because it ignores height, it fails to distinguish between short children with adequate body weight and tall, thin children. It also requires exact knowledge of children's ages. However, weight-for-age can be useful in following individual children over time, to monitor a child's development, or to identify a downward trend (although it is not possible to be certain whether a downward trend is due to linear growth retardation, wasting, or both).

Height-for-age

Height-for-age — comparison of a child's height or length with the reference median height for children of the same age and sex — is also of limited value for nutritional screening or assessment surveys in nutritional emergencies. Stunting indicates a slowing in skeletal growth, and, since linear growth responds very slowly compared with weight, it tends to reflect long-standing nutritional inadequacy, repeated infections, and poor overall economic and/or environmental conditions.

Height-for-age assessment in children under 5 years has proved useful in refugee populations for monitoring nutritional well-being in the long term (i.e. over a number of years) once wasting malnutrition has been controlled.

Arm circumference

Measurements of mid-upper arm circumference (MUAC) provide an alternative means for nutritional screening of children from 6 months to 5 years of age. They are useful when resources are limited and where weight and height measurements cannot be done; however, arm circumference measurements are inaccurate and open to several criticisms:

- Measuring techniques are difficult to standardize and results vary widely both within and between observers. This variation may not be eliminated even with careful training, and in emergency situations the training is often less than optimal.
- The inherent measuring error is large (±1 cm) and the difference between −2 SD and −3 SD is not much more than 1 cm. Consequently, many children may be wrongly classified (false-positives = children classed as malnourished who are not; false-negatives = malnourished children who are passed as normal).
- Perhaps most important of all, there is normally an increase in arm circumference of about 2 cm between 6 months and 5 years of age. When a single cut-off is applied, there will inevitably be some distortion, i.e. some normal children aged 1–2 years will be classed as malnourished (which is perhaps not important) while some aged 3–4 years will be classed as normal when they are in fact malnourished.

In circumstances in which weight or height cannot be measured, but where ages are known or can be estimated (e.g. from calendars of local events) with reasonable accuracy, one feasible solution to these problems is determination of MUAC-for-age. Reference values are given in Table A3.4. An alternative is to measure MUAC-for-length (or MUAC-for-height); Table A3.5 gives reference values. These tables include values for boys and girls together, for use when sex differentiation is impracticable. Suitable equipment is described in Annex 3 and consists of either a QUAC stick (for MUAC-for-height) or a length-measuring board marked with the cut-offs corresponding to median −2 SD (values for boys on one side, girls on the other). If the QUAC stick is used, care must be taken to include all children up to 110 cm in height (or from 60 to 100 cm in growth-retarded populations); it is therefore necessary, but difficult, to measure the height of all children aged from birth to 2 years. The length board marked with MUAC value is preferable. Table 19 illustrates the interpretation of MUAC values.

Interpretation of different indices

When data on wasting (weight-for-height) are compared with those for weight-for-age or height-for-age, it must be borne in mind that a given deficit in weight-

Table 19 *Examples of MUAC[a] cut-off points for classifying malnourished children*

Nutritional status	Standard deviations (SD) below reference median MUAC
Well nourished and mild PEM	Equal to or above −2 SD
Moderate PEM	Below −2 SD, equal to or above −3 SD
Severe PEM	Below −3 SD

[a] MUAC-for age or MUAC-for-height.

Table 20 *Classification of severity of malnutrition in a community, based on the prevalence of wasting and mean weight-for-height Z-score, for children under 5 years of age*

Severity of malnutrition	Prevalence of wasting (% below median −2 SD)	Mean weight-for-height Z-score
Acceptable	<5%	>−0.40
Poor	5–9%	−0.40 to −0.69
Serious	10–14%	−0.70 to −0.99
Critical	≥15%	≤−1.00

for-height (e.g. Z-score −2) is of much greater physiological significance than a similar deficit in weight-for-age or height-for-age. For instance, a population of whom 10% are below −2 SD weight-for-height has serious acute undernutrition; but if 10% are below −2 SD weight-for-age, the associated risks are lower. Table 20 provides guidance on interpreting weight-for-height prevalence rates in terms of Z-score cut-offs (−2 SD weight-for-height, and mean Z-score).

Older age groups

While the nutritional status of children under 5 years is of primary concern in most situations — and can be taken to reflect the nutritional status of the whole community — older children, adolescents, and adults also suffer when there are food shortages. Indeed, in cultures where the feeding of young children has precedence over that of the parents, it may be school-age children, adolescents, or adults who are most affected by a lack of food.

Weight-for-height can easily be assessed in children of school age using similar tables to those for children of preschool age. However, the curves for median −2 SD and 80% of reference median weight-for-height do not run parallel in any population and it is therefore essential to use the Z-score system. With this proviso, data for school-age children can be very useful in providing a more complete picture of the nutritional status of the community. However, the age at which the growth spurt of adolescence occurs is variable, and it is difficult to adjust both for this and for sexual maturity. Therefore, only children up to 10 years of age should be considered.

In individuals aged over 19 years, BMI can be used in conjunction with clinical assessments, where BMI = (weight in kg)/(height in metres)^2.

BMI cut-off points adopted by WHO for various levels of thinness are given in Table A3.6 of Annex 3.

Adults are assessed as being severely malnourished if they have bilateral oedema not attributable to other causes (such as renal disease, anaemia, beriberi, liver disease, or varicose veins) or if they are extremely thin. Thinness is assessed from measurements of body weight and height by reference to Table A3.6. If the body weight is below the figure given in the column for BMI 16 for that person's height, it signifies severe thinness or wasting. If actual body weight is between the values for BMI 16.0 and 17.0, the individual is classed as moderately thin or wasted, and if it is between the values for BMI 17.0 and 18.5, it signifies marginal thinness. The same cut-offs apply to both sexes and to elderly people.

Surveys of adults, even on a limited scale, can be most useful in helping to determine whether a whole population is affected by undernutrition or whether young children are more affected. In the latter case, the malnutrition is probably related more to feeding practices or to common infections among children than to overall food shortage.

Clinical and other indicators of malnutrition

There are a number of clinical signs of protein–energy malnutrition or specific nutritional deficiencies that can be rapidly assessed by examining a child and that require no instruments or tests:

- *Oedema*. In extreme situations or where kwashiorkor is the prevalent form of malnutrition, simple surveys (or screening) for oedema may be sufficiently precise to confirm a severe problem, and body measurements may be unnecessary. Depending on the local situation, it may be appropriate to look for oedema of the feet, especially in young children. Oedema of the feet can also occur in adult populations, especially pregnant or lactating women and elderly people.
- *Clinical marasmus* (if a standardized clinical definition is applied).
- *Night blindness*, revealed by questioning mothers, or *eye signs* of xerophthalmia (vitamin A deficiency).
- *Extreme pallor* in severe anaemia.
- *Selected clinical signs of other vitamin or mineral deficiencies* of potential local importance, depending on the basic diet of the population (see Chapter 2).

Such clinical signs are valuable as indicators and may be sufficient when resources are limited. However, observations by different people are not easily comparable and standardization is very difficult; they are also imprecise. For example, oedema or clinical signs of marasmus will fail to identify many severely malnourished individuals. Anthropometry is also needed for individual monitoring.

The following information is also important and relevant to assessment of acute malnutrition:

- *Incidence of diseases associated with PEM*, including measles, diarrhoea (defined, for instance, as three or more loose stools per day), and whooping cough.
- *Mortality data*, since PEM is associated with increased mortality in young children (e.g. from measles).

In all cases, the data collected should be expressed as rates, over a specified time period. Mortality rates are usually expressed per ten thousand, e.g. the daily mortality rate (per ten thousand) in a refugee camp or definable area is:

$$\frac{\text{average number of deaths in the camp or area per day}}{\text{total number of people in the camp or area}} \times 10000$$

Thus, if there are 14 deaths in a week (7 days) among a population of 5000, the daily mortality rate is:

$$\left[(14/7) \times 10000\right]/5000 = 4 \text{ per } 10000 \text{ per day}$$

Using body measurement indicators

Techniques for measuring weight, height, and arm circumference, and for selecting children under 5 years of age or less than 100 cm in height[1] are described in Annex 3.

Reference values for weight-for-height are also given in Annex 3. To classify the nutritional status of a child, the child's weight is compared with the values given opposite his or her height, yielding the Z-score (SD) range in which the child falls. Separate tables are provided for girls and boys and for the sexes combined (Tables A3.1 and A3.2). If a personal computer is to be used, software is available for analysis of anthropometric data (e.g. EpiInfo[2]). At most ages, girls have significantly lower weight-for-length or weight-for-height than boys. Using the "unisex" table therefore implies a systematic error, with slightly increased rates of underweight status for girls and the selection of slightly too many girls when the table is used for screening purposes.

In practice, surveys and many screening operations focus on children under 5 years of age (0–59 months). This is because, in most societies, young children are the most vulnerable to malnutrition in food emergencies, and their nutritional status is a good indicator of that of the population as a whole. If children's ages are not known precisely, and it is difficult to ascertain which are under 5 years, an acceptable procedure is to examine only those children who are below 100 cm in height (the approximate mean height of children aged 5 years in a stunted population).[3]

Classification of malnutrition

Body measurements give reasonably accurate estimates of body wasting. Children more than 3 SD below the median reference weight-for-height can be said with some certainty to be severely malnourished, while those between 2 and

[1] In populations not previously chronically undernourished (and therefore not stunted) the cut-off should be 110 cm, which is the median reference height of children aged 5 years.

[2] A list of distributors can be obtained from Expanded Programme on Immunization, World Health Organization, 1211 Geneva 27, Switzerland.

[3] Surveys may be based on children aged 0–59, 6–59, or 12–59 months. Whichever lower age limit is chosen, it is essential that the same limit be applied in all surveys, whether among different populations or in subsequent surveys among the same population. If different limits/criteria are applied, the results will not be comparable. It is more difficult to make accurate measurements on children less than 6–12 months, and their status may differ significantly from that of older children.

3 SD below the median are moderately malnourished. However, of the children not yet below −2 SD, some may also be malnourished in reality, particularly in communities where more than 15% of the population have weight-for-height values less than 2 SD below the reference median.

Table 18 shows weight-for-height cut-offs for classification into two or three nutritional groups. For most purposes — e.g. identifying those individuals who need therapeutic feeding, those who need supplementary feeding, and those who need no special, selective feeding — three groups (defined by two cut-off points) are appropriate. If the availability of food is a major (but potentially short-term) constraint, the cut-off points may have to be defined on the basis of a pilot survey, in such a way that the children are classified according to the food available to feed them.

Table 19 shows typical MUAC cut-offs for classifying malnourished children. It should be noted that there is no exact equivalence between the different indicators: each method will result in slightly different prevalences in each classification and consequently different "rates" of malnutrition. Nonetheless, consistent use of one method over a period of time will provide a reasonable estimate of nutritional conditions and trends.

Arm circumference should be used only when circumstances make it impossible to use weight-for-height measurement, or as a preliminary screening procedure before measuring weight-for-height.

Rapid nutritional surveys

A rapid survey is normally undertaken as part of the initial assessment to obtain an overview of the nutritional situation, identify any particular nutritional problems, and determine which areas and population groups are worst affected. In most situations, surveys should be repeated periodically — every 3 months during the initial stages, if possible — to monitor changes over time. In all cases, surveys must be carefully planned and managed, otherwise the results will be unreliable and probably misleading.

Most nutritional surveys in emergencies focus on determining the nutritional status of children under 5 years (see page 42), which is a good indicator of that of the community as a whole. In practice, it may be convenient to survey only children up to 100 cm in length or height. It is also advantageous to assess the nutritional status of adults directly, using body mass index; if adults are also malnourished, this strengthens the case for general food distribution (see Chapter 4). If adults are not malnourished, it is likely that child feeding practices or recurrent infections may be playing a major role in the high rates of malnutrition among young children, or the children may be suffering from micronutrient malnutrition rather than PEM.

The following steps are essential in planning and organizing a nutritional survey:

- defining the objectives and data required
- determining sample size
- specifying the indicators and sampling methods to be used

- designing and pretesting data collection forms and analysis sheets
- gathering the necessary equipment
- selecting and training survey personnel
- scheduling and conducting fieldwork under supervision
- analysing, interpreting, and reporting the findings
- determining the implications of the findings for action — policy decisions and intervention activities.

The various kinds of survey results that might be obtained, and the actions that may be needed, should be imaginatively envisaged from the planning stage. This forethought should influence the timing and geographical scope of the survey, the age groups and sampling methods, etc., and the presentation and interpretation of results. Community leaders should be involved throughout the process. The purpose of the exercise should be explained to them and their cooperation sought.

The validity and usefulness of the results depend on the consistent application of proper sampling procedures, the accuracy of measurements and recording, and a clear, prompt presentation of the findings; the justification for the whole procedure is the immediate use to which the results should be put.

Objectives and data required

The purposes of the survey, the populations to be surveyed,[1] and the specific uses to be made of the data must be clearly defined at the outset and agreed by all concerned. The information to be collected on individuals and households can then be specified as follows:

- Body measurements indicating nutritional status — usually weight and height, possibly arm circumference — and the presence of oedema. These details represent the minimum necessary information. In emergencies, children are normally classified according to the cut-offs shown in Table 11. Where more detail is required, and feasible, classification may be based on intervals of 1 standard deviation below the median, or intervals of 10% or 5% below the reference value.
- Specific location (village or camp sector) and/or membership of a particular population subgroup. This information may be important for comparing different groups and thus targeting assistance. (A representative sample must then be drawn from each group separately.)
- Supplementary information that might be useful. This includes: age; sex; length of time in current location (for refugees or displaced persons); measles immunization status; recent deaths in the household; availability of cooking utensils and fuel; food distributions already made; occurrence of clinical cases of anaemia, xerophthalmia, beriberi, etc. in nearby health centres or hospitals.

When a rapid determination of current nutritional status is necessary and resources are limited, data collection should be restricted to body measurements

[1] Depending on the situation, the population might be defined as children, specific cultural or economic groups, all refugees in a particular location, etc.

among specifically identified population groups. Even when it is agreed (and feasible) to gather additional data at the same time, these should be limited to a few details that are easily measured or classified, and on which action can be taken.[1]

Indicators and sampling methods to be used

For weight-for-height measurements the choice and systematic application of an appropriate sampling method are crucial. Annex 4 provides detailed information on the statistical procedures involved. "Random" or "systematic" sampling methods should be used if reliable and up-to-date registers are available, or the area is small and orderly. Otherwise, two-stage cluster sampling is advisable. Personnel with experience in field surveys and statistical analysis may be able to help and advise; if not, a reasonable "rule of thumb" is to select a minimum of 450 children for random sampling and a minimum of 30 clusters for cluster sampling.[2] Thirty children should be measured in each cluster, following the procedures described in Annex 4 to select both the clusters and the children within each chosen cluster. Annex 4 provides guidelines on sample sizes and on drawing a random sample.

Data collection forms and analysis sheets

Examples of two very different survey data collection forms are presented in Figs 5 and 6. A form of the type shown in Fig. 5 would be suitable for use in a rapid survey designed to obtain a simple, crude estimate of levels of malnutrition in particular localities, for instance in a rapid assessment mission. Each child measured is represented by a tick or stroke in the appropriate box. When all children in the selected sample have been measured, the number of ticks in each box is counted, and percentages calculated. Recording is quick and easy, but there is no possibility of cross-checking later for any errors.

Note: The sample size for systematic random sampling is 450 children where the total number of households is less than 10 000. In a small population (2000–3000 people), all eligible children should be examined. The minimum sample size for cluster sampling is 30 clusters of 30 children (i.e. 900 children).

A form similar to that in Fig. 6 could be used when a few additional items of information are to be collected and cross-tabulations made between different items. One line would be completed for each child measured and interviewed; a separate form would be used for each locality or cluster. Forms of this type have been widely used in surveys among refugee populations.

Alternatively, a form such as that shown in Fig. 7 can be designed for recording the personal details and required data on each child individually. This particular form includes a dietary-recall question on infant/young child and family feed-

---

[1] Data items, such as the presence of anaemia, based on clinical observations should *not* be included: the estimates would vary from one enumerator to another and be unreliable. Evidence of deficiencies of vitamin A or vitamin C should be included only if all observers have similar and adequate experience in such assessments.

[2] Clusters are the smallest possible distinct geographical subdivisions within the total area or population of interest, e.g. a village, section of a camp, or geographical area delimited by a road or river.

Fig. 5 Data collection form: simple tabulation of weight-for-length and oedema for children up to 110 cm in length (100 cm if growth-retarded)

Length	Number examined[a]	Weight-for-length below median −Z		With bilateral oedema			
				Below median −2Z		Above median −2Z	
		Number	%[b]	Number	%[b]	Number	%[b]
<85 cm[c] (<24 months)	⧄⧄⧄⧄⧄⊓ ⧄⧄⧄⧄⧄ 53	⧄ ⧄ 10	18.9	⊓ 3	5.7	| 1	1.9
85–110 cm (24–59 months)	⧄⧄⧄⧄⧄⧄┌ ⧄⧄⧄⧄⧄⧄ 62	⧄□ ⧄ 14	22.6	| 1	1.6	⊓ 3	4.8
Total sample	115	24	20.9	4	3.5	4	3.5

[a] Numbers of subjects in each "box" are tallied using strokes, or lines forming a small box; 3 subjects would be recorded as / / / or ⊓, and five as ~~////~~ or ⧄, and so on.

[b] Percentage of the whole sample in the age category concerned.

[c] 82–83 cm in growth-retarded populations.

ing, which enables a rapid assessment to be made of dietary practices. Personnel can also be trained to make this a quantitative recall method.[1] It also includes a summary of recent illnesses, which is useful in assessing the contribution of infections to malnutrition. Such a survey, of course, reflects only the situation at the time; the situation is liable to change rapidly, as the emergency evolves and even as the seasons change. A separate form, similar to that in Fig. 6, is then needed to summarize the data and facilitate their analysis (unless data are entered directly into a computer for analysis).

Forms must be prepared in a language which is fully understood by the personnel who will collect the data, and should be pilot-tested by such personnel. The layout, language, and explanatory notes must be refined to minimize any possibility of misunderstandings or errors in recording. The more data are to be collected and the more complex the form, the more time will be required to develop and test the form, determine the necessary sample size, and train survey personnel.

Equipment

The following supplies and equipment will be needed by each team carrying out a weight-for-height survey:

— 2 hanging spring scales (see Annex 3 for description) with several sets of pants and a basket or cradle for infants (and spare scale), or a beam-balance scale with basket

— support (tripod, pole, etc.) for scale

— height-measuring stick and platform

[1] *Field guide on rapid nutritional assessment in emergencies.* Alexandria, WHO Regional Office for the Eastern Mediterranean, 1995.

Fig. 6 Example of a more detailed group data collection form

Cluster no. ....
Date of survey ..../..../....
Birth date before which children should be measured standing (height) rather than lying (length) ..../..../....

Village/section ....
District ....
Team no. ....

No.	Name of child (optional)	Age[a] (m)	Sex M = 1 F = 2	Weight[b] (kg)	Height[b] (cm)	Oedema	Arm circ. (cm)	Var. 1[c]	Var. 2[c]	Var. 3[c]	Var. 4[c]
1				.	.						
2				.	.						
3				.	.						
4				.	.						
5				.	.						
6				.	.						
7				.	.						
8				.	.						
9				.	.						
10				.	.						
11				.	.						
12				.	.						
13				.	.						
14				.	.						
15				.	.						
16				.	.						
17				.	.						
18				.	.						
19				.	.						
20				.	.						
21				.	.						
22				.	.						
23				.	.						
24				.	.						
25				.	.						
26				.	.						
27				.	.						
28				.	.						
29				.	.						
30				.	.						

[a] Age (completed months) should be determined from birth certificate if possible, otherwise by constructing a calendar of known local or national events and identifying the nearest such event to the birth of the child.

[b] Enter the weight and length (if < 85 cm) or height (if ≥ 85 cm) with one decimal figure, e.g. 10.5 kg, 73.2 cm.

[c] Other variables, if available, may be entered here, such as clinical anaemia, xerophthalmia, spleen enlargement, diarrhoea, dehydration.

Fig. 7 Nutrition and health survey form for children under 5 years

A. *General*

Date ..../..../.... Village .... Serial no. ....

	Family name	First name
Child	....	....
Mother	....	....
Father	....	....

Child's date of birth ..../..../.....
Age (months) ....

No. of children born alive to this mother ....
(complete this question only once for each mother)
No. of her children still living ....

B. *Feeding of child and family (the previous day)*
Breast-feeding of child Yes/No

	Child		Family	
Time of day	Foods given	Method of cooking	Foods consumed	Method of cooking
Morning				
Midday				
Evening				
Snacks: Morning Afternoon Evening				

C. *Clinical history and examination*

		Yes	No
Yesterday, did the child have:	fever	( )	( )
	cough	( )	( )
	diarrhoea	( )	( )
In the past 3 months, has the child had:	measles	( )	( )
	other (specify)		
Does the child now have:	oedema	( )	( )
	anaemia (pallor)	( )	( )

Child's weight ..... kg Length ..... cm MUAC ..... cm
Remarks:
Signature of person examining:

— height/length board (length 120 cm for children <5 years, or 150 cm if all children are included)

— set of known weights to check accuracy of scales

— clipboard, pencils, and erasers

— data collection forms (as in Fig. 5, 6, or 7)

— weight-for-height reference tables for boys and girls separately (Table A3.1)

— tables of body mass index for adults (Table A3.6) if they are measured

— pocket calculator and/or notebook computer

— table and chairs

— vehicle and fuel.

A number of saftware packages have been developed by WHO and the Centers for Disease Control and Prevention which are valuable for the statistical analysis of both epidemiological data in general (e.g. EpiInfo) and anthropometric data (e.g. EPINUT, ANTHRO).

Survey personnel: selection and training

Local personnel should be recruited and trained to carry out the surveys. Each survey team should have two or three members, one of whom may also serve as the driver, and should be able to weigh and measure up to 200 children in an assembled group in a single location in one day. When a survey is based on cluster sampling, a team might be able to complete two, or possibly three, clusters per day. There should be enough teams to complete all data collection within 2–3 days.

One supervisor should be available for every two or three teams; he or she should participate in training and monitor the data collection work in the field.

At least 4 days should be allowed to train personnel who have no previous experience in measuring children. Training should provide plenty of practice in measuring children in a calm setting before a real survey is undertaken. Team members, working together, should practise: selecting samples; weighing and measuring children (to ensure consistency and comparability between individuals and teams); collecting other required information; and recording everything accurately on data collection forms.[1]

Organizing fieldwork

Fieldwork must be planned in close consultation with the leaders of the communities concerned, avoiding special days when other important activities occur, such as food distributions or religious festivals. The overall schedule should allow sufficient time for preparation, training, community mobilization, reporting, and data analysis.

Every effort must be made to ensure proper sampling methods and accuracy in measuring and recording. Supervisors must be mobile so that they can verify sampling procedures and make spot-checks on measurements carried out by the teams for which they are responsible.

Analysis, interpretation, and reporting of survey results

The data obtained from a sample survey provide only an estimate of the true malnutrition rate in a population. Data can be analysed and the results presented in terms of either standard deviations or percentages. Standard deviations are more appropriate but for people with little background in statistics percentages are more easily understood and calculated, and are therefore more widely used, particularly in emergencies. The "confidence interval" for the data (see Annex 4) should be calculated and reported whenever possible.

The data should ideally be classified by one-year age groups (12–23 months, 24–35 months, etc.) or by height ranges, to identify any significant differences and

---

[1] A good method for checking and comparing the accuracy and reliability of team members in making measurements (weight and height) is given in Annex 1 of *Measuring change in nutritional status* (Geneva, World Health Organization, 1983).

pinpoint the children at particularly high risk within the under-5 age group. These data should be summarized and presented as in Fig. 8. This information can then be used to try to improve the targeting of feeding programmes and/or as a basis for appropriate health and community education measures. Guidelines for interpreting weight-for-height data are given in Table 20 (page 40).

A statistically more sensitive way of analysing the data is to express the results as the mean and standard error of the mean of the individual indices (weight-for-height expressed as a percentage of, or in terms of Z-scores below, the median of the reference population). For instance, the mean weight-for-height may be 90 ± 2% that of the reference population. This method of analysis allows more sensitive comparisons to be made between different population groups or of a series of measurements over time in a given population. For practical purposes, calculation of mean Z-scores requires computer facilities.

Children more than 3 SD below the reference value of weight-for-height, or below 70% of that value, or with oedema are at high risk of death and need immediate therapeutic feeding and medical care. Survey teams must be able to refer such cases for immediate treatment.

Once survey results have been tabulated, a concise summary report should be prepared, which should include a brief description of the methodology (e.g. sampling), the results, and interpretation, plus practical recommendations for action. The report should not be delayed while detailed analyses of the data are awaited, especially if urgent decisions on relief activities have to be made.

Care is essential in making comparisons between data from different surveys. For instance:

- Whether or not different "percentages wasted" are significant has to be assessed statistically, as described above and in Annex 3.

Fig. 8 Example of a data summary sheet for the presentation of community data[a]

Age	No. of subjects	Weight-for-height (W/H)		Total W/H prevalence below median −2Z	Mean of W/H Z-scores, and SEM[b]	% with oedema	
		% below median −3Z	% below median −2Z but equal to or above median −3Z			below median −2Z	equal to or above median −2Z
6–11 m 0–11 m							
12–17 m 18–23 m 12–23 m							
24–35 m 36–47 m 48–59 m 24–59 m							
0–59 m							
5–9.9 y							

[a] Form should be prepared for boys, for girls, and for the sexes combined.
[b] Standard error of the mean.

- Illnessess (diarrhoeal diseases, measles, malaria, etc.) may have as important an influence as food supply/availability.
- Feeding practices, e.g. food distribution within the family, may be equally important.
- Previous food distribution may have significantly altered the situation.
- The child population examined may not be properly representative, e.g. seriously ill children may not be brought for examination because carers do not wish to expose them.
- In the same population much higher prevalences of malnutrition are often found for narrower age ranges, for example between 12 and 24 months.
- In populations who are already malnourished, or in a very severe famine, much higher prevalences may be seen which, for the purpose of setting relief priorities, might need additional classification.
- If prevalences are lower than would be expected from the severity of the emergency, the possibility that many children have already died must be considered.
- Immediate relief action can be linked to the levels of prevalence found, keeping in mind the available resources.

Additional factors to bear in mind are indicated in the section on nutritional surveillance (page 54).

Individual screening

Individual children (and sometimes adults) are selected by screening for admission to selective — supplementary and/or therapeutic — feeding programmes if the assessment has shown that such programmes are needed and the necessary resources are available. *All* the potentially eligible individuals in the target population groups must be screened.

Screening is usually done intermittently to select individuals for specific nutritional assistance during a predetermined period. Selected individuals (or families) are registered and given cards that entitle them to food at several subsequent distributions (see Chapter 4). In some cases, screening may be done on each occasion that food is distributed.

The following steps are essential in planning and organizing a screening exercise:

- specifying the objectives, method, and criteria to be used
- specifying who is to be screened
- gathering the necessary equipment and arranging transport
- selecting and training personnel
- scheduling the screening.

Objectives, methods, and criteria

The purpose of the screening exercise must be clearly defined and understood by all concerned. The approach, and particularly the number of separate classification categories required, will be determined by the overall situation and the responses — and by the resources available. When there are, say, four possible courses of action (e.g. no assistance, weekly ration, daily ration, or intensive supervised feeding), four categories should be established.

Realistic selection criteria (i.e. cut-off points) must be set. For instance, there is little point in selecting a large number of malnourished children unless facilities are available and can be organized to provide them with appropriate assistance.

Weight-for-height should be used for the screening itself whenever possible. Children with oedema should be identified and automatically classified as severely malnourished. However, if a very large number of young children have to be screened and categorized quickly, with few staff and little equipment, the simple MUAC method should be used, at least initially, with appropriate cut-off points.

Sometimes, screening in a large population is done in two stages. In the first stage, MUAC is measured in all children aged 1–5 years. All those with MUAC below median −2 SD for age or for length, plus any obviously malnourished older children, should be referred for weighing. The second stage involves weight-for-height assessments of all those referred.

It is also important to specify any additional, clinical criteria (such as obvious sickness or signs or symptoms of serious disease) for the classification — and registration for assistance — of children and of other vulnerable groups, such as pregnant or lactating women.

Screening is *not* a survey procedure. Nevertheless, for continuing surveillance purposes, periodic screening can provide valuable data for monitoring trends in the situation.

Who is to be screened

The populations to be screened must be clearly defined. This will depend upon the local situation, and it is essential to remember that people attending relief centres are not necessarily the worst affected. Malnourished individuals may remain at home, because they are unable to walk, live in relatively inaccessible areas, or, in the case of marasmic children or those with kwashiorkor, are not regarded by their parents as being in need of help.

Personnel and equipment

A team of six workers, given one day of appropriate training, can screen from 500 to 2000 individuals a day (but fewer in sparsely populated areas).

The equipment needed for each measuring team is essentially the same as that for surveys (page 48), plus:

— 2 tape-measures (ideally of fibreglass or locally made), if MUAC is to be measured

— QUAC stick (Fig. A3.5) or, preferably, length-board showing MUAC cut-offs (median −2 SD)
— tables of MUAC-for-age (Table A3.4) or MUAC-for-length (Table A3.5)
— registration books and ration cards for each category of selected beneficiary
— 2 rubber date-stamps and one official stamp to validate the ration cards (important for preventing abuses).

The pocket calculator and vehicle/fuel may not be needed for regular screening procedures.

Procedure: organizing screening sessions

The community should be informed, through local leaders, at least 24 hours in advance of a screening session to allow them to arrange for eligible people to attend. The time chosen for the session should be convenient for the community.

When large numbers of people are to be screened careful organization is essential; those awaiting screening should be seated, preferably out of the sun. Existing buildings should be used as screening locations whenever possible. It may be useful to erect temporary barriers to channel people to and from the places where measurements are made.

Severely malnourished individuals should be selected first by clinical examination. If people are well organized, this can be done very quickly by an experienced individual walking along the rows of waiting people. Severely ill people must not be kept waiting for long periods of time.

A system of individual identification should be used, such as date-stamping the ration card or marking the individual's fingernail with a 10% silver nitrate solution. It is important that each individual understands what is being done and why. If food is to be distributed immediately as the direct result of a screening, the selected individuals should be shown to the appropriate distribution point.

When whole communities are screened, results should be recorded in terms of the total population and the numbers of individuals assigned to different categories. These records can be useful for making comparisons with future screening or survey results. Other observations, including the presence of oedema, should also be recorded.

Nutritional surveillance

The purpose of nutritional surveillance is to detect changes in the nutritional status of a population over a period of time. A continuing surveillance system in areas prone to disaster (e.g. drought) will greatly facilitate assessments in any future disaster. It will also indicate when an intervention such as supplementary feeding may be phased out, and help to ensure that there is no subsequent relapse into malnutrition. Surveillance involves the systematic collection and analysis of:

• data from periodic nutritional surveys

- results of periodic screening
- reports from supplementary and therapeutic feeding centres and health clinics
- morbidity and mortality data.

Information on food distributions and on developments in such areas as agricultural production and employment among the affected populations should also be collected and considered in parallel with nutritional data.

Periodic nutritional surveys

A comparison of nutritional survey results obtained at different times will show trends in the nutritional status of a population. However, valid comparison requires the use of standardized survey methods and sampling techniques (see Annex 4).

Baseline data indicating the usual nutritional status of the population are important as a basis for comparison, but may not always be available at the beginning of an emergency. Comparisons between data from successive surveys can reveal whether nutritional status is worsening or improving, and can help in evaluation of the effectiveness of food and nutrition relief operations. A measure of variance (SD or standard error of the mean) of each successive survey is therefore desirable, so that the statistical significance of apparent differences between populations, or within the same population over time, can be assessed.

Comparisons between several sets of measurements taken at different times from the same community must be interpreted with caution. Many severely malnourished children die in nutritional emergencies, leaving fewer children to be counted as malnourished in later surveys. A declining malnutrition rate may thus be due to a high death rate among the severely malnourished rather than to any improvement in the nutritional situation. Similarly, improvements in nutritional conditions *in spite of* an inefficient food relief programme might be the result of seasonal or economic factors.

The findings of a series of surveys should always be compared with mortality data gathered between survey dates and with other available information (such as morbidity data, especially in epidemics) relevant to health and socioeconomic conditions.

Periodic screenings

Body measurement data collected during periodic screenings of vulnerable groups (for eligibility for special food assistance) can be used to produce "nutritional profiles" of the populations screened. These profiles *may* indicate whether the proportion of malnourished individuals is changing, and in what way. However, even small differences in the procedure used during screening may result in different groups of people attending. A screening held early in the morning is likely to attract a different group from a screening held at midday, because people are engaged in different activities. Resulting variations can be large and can give rise to erroneous conclusions. Moreover, if only a part of the population is screened it is unlikely to be representative of the whole population.

Systematic checking of indicators other than body measurements during screening can also provide useful data, provided that they are interpreted with due care. Data may include oedema rates and signs of specific mineral and vitamin deficiencies. Because organization of screening sessions is likely to take up considerable amounts of time, several such indicators should be checked during each session whenever possible.

Records from supplementary and therapeutic feeding centres and health clinics

Data collected weekly at selective feeding centres, fixed health facilities, and maternal and child health centres — such as the number of individuals attending for health care or nutritional relief and the nature of their problems — can give a rough idea of change in the nutritional health of the affected population and particular vulnerable groups. Such data should be used with caution: they are not wholly representative, although they can provide an indication of changes that may be occurring in the overall population. They do, however, give a good picture of which members of the population feel they need nutritional attention, for whatever reason, and are physically able to attend nutrition clinics (e.g. live within walking distance).

Local auxiliary personnel can be recruited and trained to gather data for the surveillance of simple signs and symptoms of malnutrition at village or camp level. Training might be organized as follows:

- 1 day: major signs of PEM (wasting, oedema)
  investigation of anaemia and night blindness
  diagnosis of major eye lesions due to vitamin A deficiency
  clinical signs of other mineral and vitamin deficiencies
  organizing the collection of information.
- 1 day: practice in measuring weight (and/or arm circumference) and height, and recording, analysing, interpreting, and reporting results.
- 1 day: field test; a simple survey — data collection, analysis, presentation.

Health surveillance

Apart from the strictly nutritional data gathered by surveillance, there is both an initial and a continuing need for health information of a broader nature. In emergencies affecting large and stable populations much of this information may already be available, but for newly created communities, such as those of refugees and displaced persons, a broad needs assessment is generally required, followed by the establishment of a new health information system.

The initial assessment must first establish the population that is affected — the number of people and their location and living conditions. This is necessary both for the proper planning of rations and other services and facilities, and for calculating mortality rate, which is an important indicator of the adequacy of any rehabilitation programme. Methods of assessment include the following:

- Ideally, census or registration of individuals on arrival in a location. This is not always feasible, and information requires periodic updating.

- Aerial photography combined with household surveys to estimate the average number of people and their age distribution (in 5-year brackets) per house/ shelter.
- Mapping of camps and estimation of total population by identifying zones of high, medium, and low density, and counting the people in several squares (e.g. 100 m × 100 m) in each zone.
- In an immunization programme, counting the number of children under 5 years of age immunized. Estimating the percentage coverage in the community allows the number of children under 5 years and — by extrapolation — the total population to be estimated.

CHAPTER 4

Nutritional relief: general feeding programmes

General feeding programmes provide food to the affected population as a whole. If the population is entirely dependent upon external aid, the general ration must provide for a minimum intake of 2100 $kcal_{th}$ per person per day, and more if the population is malnourished, exposed to cold, or does heavy physical work. The general ration is normally provided dry, for people to cook at home. Distribution of cooked meals to large populations should be considered only when there is no alternative, for instance where there is insufficient cooking fuel and when there is a security problem.

The food commodities provided must: match the food needs and habits of the recipients; be convenient to transport, store, and distribute; and be equitably distributed. Where the population does not have cooking utensils or fuel, these must be provided. Arrangements must also be made for the milling of whole-grain cereals.

Good organization and coordination between all concerned is the key to the success of a food distribution operation. The effectiveness of all feeding programmes should be monitored at regular intervals.

Introduction

A general feeding programme is required when the population does not have access to sufficient food to meet its nutritional needs. Ensuring an adequate basic ration for the affected population is of utmost importance at the onset of an emergency. Providing rations that satisfy the full nutritional needs of the population largely avoids the need for additional selective food distribution programmes, which are logistically more difficult, as well as more costly and time-consuming, to organize. If an adequate ration is not provided, some children are likely to develop signs of malnutrition. Prevention is always better than cure. The ability of the population to provide a part of their needs from other sources, on a sustainable basis, should be carefully assessed, and the general rations should be adjusted to make up the difference.

A selective feeding programme, by contrast, targets the most nutritionally vulnerable groups through supplementary feeding, and those in need of nutritional rehabilitation through therapeutic feeding; this is discussed in Chapter 5. In nutritional emergencies, women, young children, and the elderly are particularly vulnerable. In general, it is recommended that selective food rations be provided through maternal and child health services rather than together with general rations. However, large, blanket selective feeding programmes are often used to supplement an inadequate general ration, in which case it is the general ration, rather than the blanket selective feeding ration, that should be improved.

General principles

In a population affected by an emergency, the general ration should meet the population's minimum energy, protein, fat, and micronutrient requirements for light physical activity. Where the population is exposed to cold the ration may have to be increased (see Table A1.3). Population-based averages do not meet every individual's needs; some individuals require more, others less, than the average.

Besides being nutritionally balanced, the general ration should be culturally acceptable, fit for human consumption, and easily digestible for children and other affected vulnerable groups.

Although there is a difference between the needs of a young child and those of an active adult, providing different rations to different age groups is not feasible in an operation serving a large population. The same general ration components should be provided for each person, regardless of age; families will divide the ration among themselves.

In some cases, the affected population may not be dependent on food assistance alone but may have or acquire access to some other sources of food. Food rations should then be adjusted and complement any food that the affected population is able to obtain for itself, through activities such as agricultural production, trade, labour, and small businesses. An understanding of the various mechanisms used by the population to obtain access to food is essential and makes possible a better estimate of food and nutritional needs.

The following points are important to note:

- Assisting people in their home communities is always preferable to establishing relief camps.
- Where a population depends upon food rations for most or all of its food needs, it is best to distribute rations in dry form to be cooked at home. Distribution of cooked food to large populations should be avoided except as a temporary measure, for example when people do not have utensils and fuel, and for security reasons.
- Each family must have adequate cooking utensils, fuel, and water to prepare food. Lack of any of these may have as much effect on nutritional status as an inadequate ration.

Factors that affect ration levels and composition

The average energy requirement of 2100 $kcal_{th}$, mentioned in Chapter 1, is the starting point for the definition of the food ration. Other considerations that determine the types and quantities of food to be supplied are:

- the level of self-sufficiency of the target beneficiaries;
- market and trading opportunities open to the beneficiaries;
- the losses inevitably incurred in food processing at household level.

Level of self-sufficiency

The ration may be reduced according to the types and quantities of food that target beneficiaries can reasonably be expected to provide for themselves from the following resources:

- Their own production, including farming, gardening, raising of poultry and other livestock, hunting and fishing. For instance, backyard gardens can rapidly produce green leafy vegetables and sweet potatoes and many of these are good sources of iron, vitamin C, carotenoids, and other minerals and vitamins.
- Cash incomes from paid employment and other income-generating opportunities (within or outside the camp, in the case of refugees or displaced persons). A part of such income should normally be available for the purchase of food from the local market and/or ration shops.

However, rations should be adjusted *only* if these opportunities for self-sufficiency are available to the population as a whole. Regular and significant seasonal variations in household food availability must also be taken into account. The final diet should be nutritionally balanced.[1]

Nutrient requirements and market and trading opportunities

Inclusion in the ration of a variety of foods, including fresh foods, is the best assurance of meeting micronutrient (vitamin and mineral) needs. Beneficiaries, including refugees, are often able to obtain fresh fruits and vegetables (and salt)

[1] Of the calories in the final diet, 10–12% should be in the form of protein and 17–20% in the form of fat.

by trade or barter. Where expert assessment reveals that most of the target beneficiaries can obtain adequate quantities of such items from their own production[1] and/or from the local market by purchase or barter, this should be taken into account in designing the ration. When this is not the case, however, it is imperative that rations include suitable quantities of fresh foods (to the extent feasible) and/or a fortified cereal blend. Moreover, where specific nutrient deficiency problems are identified, efforts to provide foods that contain the missing nutrients must be intensified.[2]

The trading activities and final diets of the beneficiaries should be monitored, and health and nutrition education should be arranged where needed. Trading of ration foods should not be condemned out of hand: it may be one way of achieving some variety in an otherwise monotonous diet. In addition, some people in both general and selective feeding programmes who are destitute and completely without other resources may have to part with some ration foods to meet other unavoidable needs, such as clothing or fuel, even at the cost of going hungry.

Food processing considerations

Losses that are an inevitable feature of the processing and preparation of particular food items at the household level should be taken into consideration. These include both quantitative losses (notably in respect of whole-grain cereals, which have to be milled or ground[3]) and losses of nutrients during cooking. Where whole-grain cereal is distributed, some may be traded by recipients to cover the cost of grinding, and this leads to significant reduction in consumption.

For practical, nutritional, and environmental reasons, it is preferable to provide flour, particularly in the early stages of emergency. If whole grains need to be provided, local milling capacity must be available, and the ration should include compensation for milling losses and costs (depending on local milling charges, in the range 10–20%) if these are borne by the recipients.

Foods for general distribution

The basic commodities in general rations are usually cereals, pulses, and edible oil. Other items such as salt, sugar, tea, and spices are intended to increase the palatability of relief foods. Spices have no direct nutritional value, but they greatly enhance the taste of other (possibly unfamiliar) foods, thus encouraging consumption and better nutrition. If a population is entirely dependent on relief, these items should be included in the general ration wherever possible, otherwise people will exchange or sell more nutritionally valuable foods to acquire them. Salt should always be adequately iodized (at least 20–40 parts per million, i.e. 20–40 mg iodine — as potassium iodate — per kg of salt) at consump-

---

[1] As a matter of policy, household or communal vegetable gardens, in particular, should be encouraged wherever feasible.

[2] As a last resort, the distribution of pharmaceutical supplements may be required. In such cases, preparations of the required vitamins and minerals must be specified by medical nutritionists. Multivitamin tablets are *not* appropriate. See Chapter 2.

[3] Extraction rates for wheat and maize are normally about 90% (10% loss), for sorghum about 80% (20% loss). Losses must be realistically estimated, not exaggerated.

tion level. It is generally obtainable within the country or from a neighbouring country. The iodine level at the factory should be much higher.[1]

Several precooked, blended cereal products and processed cereals are available from food aid donors (see Annex 5). When fresh food items are not available, cereal blends fortified with micronutrients can be used in either general or selective feeding. Where there is total dependence on relief foods, there is a risk of micronutrient deficiencies: beriberi may develop where highly milled rice is the sole staple, pellagra with maize, sorghum, or millet, and scurvy in arid or semiarid areas where fresh fruits and vegetables are scarce or unavailable. Micronutrients may be provided through blended foods in these circumstances. Recent assessments have shown that blended foods are well accepted by the whole family, so that they should not be reserved only for particular vulnerable groups.

Fortification levels for precooked, fortified, blended foods ordered by UNHCR/UNICEF/WFP are based on the *Guidelines on formulated supplementary foods for older infants and young children* of the Codex Alimentarius. The Guidelines indicate that 100g of the supplementary food should provide approximately two-thirds of the recommended daily requirements for the nutrients listed (see Annex 5). The vitamin/mineral premix developed for this purpose was referred to as UNIMIX. Since its original formulation, levels of added vitamins and minerals have been adjusted, and producers of blended foods now have their own specifications.

However, the fortification levels of these foods, originally designed for the supplementary feeding of young children, need to be better tailored to the overall nutrient needs of the whole population affected by a major emergency. In the future, the micronutrient levels should also be based on the recommended daily vitamin and mineral allowances that were revised during the Joint FAO/WHO Expert Consultation on Vitamin and Mineral Requirements held in Bangkok, 21–23 September 1998.

As an alternative to fortified blended food, the possibilities of fortifying the staple cereal (i.e. maize or wheat) at the national, district, or even local level are being researched.

Relief foods should be palatable and culturally acceptable, and fulfil nutritional requirements. It is important that the general ration includes the traditional staple food or a fully acceptable substitute. Requirements for grinding, water (for soaking and cooking), and cooking fuel must therefore also be considered. Ease of storage and distribution as well as costs should be taken into account.

Annex 5 provides further details and guidelines concerning the suitability of various commodities.

Oil is commonly included in rations, partly for cooking purposes and to improve palatability; in addition, it is a concentrated form of energy useful for the rehabilitation of all undernourished members of the household, and of severely malnourished children in particular. Both oil and sugar can provide a considerable increase in the energy density of the diet, and targeting their use to young children should be emphasized when rations are distributed.

---

[1] Advice on the iodization level needed in any particular case may be obtained from Programme of Nutrition, World Health Organization, 1211 Geneva 27, Switzerland.

Table 21 *Examples of adequate full rations providing 2100 $kcal_{th}$ per person per day for an emergency-affected population entirely reliant on food assistance*[a]

	Rations (g)				
	Type 1	Type 2	Type 3	Type 4[a]	Type 5
Commodity:					
Cereal flour/rice/bulgur	400	420	350	420	450
Pulses	60	50	100	60	50
Oil (vitamin A-fortified)	25	25	25	30	25
Canned fish/meat	—	20	—	30	—
Fortified blended foods	50	40	50	—	—
Sugar	15	—	20	20	20
Iodized salt	5	5	5	5	5
Fresh fruit/vegetables	—	—	—	—	100
Spices	—	—	—	—	—
Approx. food value:					
Energy ($kcal_{th}$)	2013	2106	2087	2092	2116
Protein (g; % of energy)	58 g; 11%	60 g; 11%	72 g; 14%	45 g; 9%	51 g; 10%
Fat (g; % of energy)[b]	43 g; 18%	47 g; 20%	43 g; 18%	38 g; 16%	41 g; 17%

[a] Reproduced, with permission, from *Guidelines for estimating food and nutritional needs in emergencies*, Geneva, Office of the United Nations High Commissioner for Refugees/World Food Programme, 1997.

Notes

1. For rations 1, 2, 3, and 5, the cereal used for the calculation is maize meal. Ration 4 has rice as a cereal. The lower percentage energy for protein is acceptable due to its higher quality; the slightly lower fat content is in line with food habits in rice-eating populations.
2. All the rations provide at least minimum quantities of energy, protein, and fat. Fresh foods (notably vegetables and fruits), condiments, and spices should also be available wherever possible.
3. Rations 1–3 provide additional quantities of various micronutrients through the inclusion of a fortified cereal blend. Fortified cereal blends are good sources of micronutrients and, when provided in the general ration, may be consumed by all members of the family. Normally, however, they are reserved for vulnerable groups for whom selective feeding is organized. Examples of cereal blends include corn–soy blend and wheat-soy blend (produced in the USA), faffa (produced in Ethiopia), and likuni phala (produced in Malawi).

When whole-grain cereals are used for general distribution, these will require milling. Where this cannot be done by each family, more general provision must be made, either through commercial mills or by providing mills in each camp. It should also be borne in mind that pulses sometimes require long hours of cooking; those that do should be avoided in areas where fuel is scarce or too expensive. Maize and sorghum rations should be supplemented by other sources of niacin, such as groundnuts. A few examples of rations that provide the standard minimum 2100 $kcal_{th}$ per person per day are given in Table 21.

Whether an average of 2100 $kcal_{th}$ per person per day is adequate or whether an enhanced energy intake is required depends on the health status of the dependent population, the level of physical activity, the climate, and the demographic composition of the population. Enhanced rations might be required when a population is more or less totally dependent on food aid rations *and* is debilitated, exposed to cold, or engaged in heavy work.

Organizing general dry ration distributions

The key to a successful food distribution programme is good organization. The following are important aspects of ensuring fair distribution:

- Each person should have some form of identification. In small populations, e.g. in villages and small camps, lists of names held at the distribution point often suffice. When large groups are involved, lists become unmanageable and family ration cards are usually required.
- Proper arrangements must be made to ensure orderly distribution, particularly for a large population. If rations are to be given out to, say, 5000 people, it is unrealistic to expect them quietly to form a queue and take food from openly exposed sacks — chaos would result. People are more likely to comply with the distribution system if they understand how it is organized and have trust in it. The recipients should always be aware of the amounts of food to which they are entitled; public information meetings should be held, as well as meetings with administrative and natural leaders.
- Spot checks should take place at distribution points to ensure that the correct ration is being distributed in the correct quantities.

It is essential that food supplies are ordered in good time. The quantity needed to feed 1000 people for 1 month is approximately 16.4 tonnes. To cover losses in transit, an additional 5% should be added in countries with a port or 10% in landlocked countries.

To eliminate personal bias, favouritism, and vulnerability to pressure, reliable individuals should be recruited from outside the community to fill responsible positions such as storekeeping and administration (see Chapter 7).

Distributing commodities by volume rather than weight is usually quicker and more accurate: accurate scales are unlikely to be available at all distribution points and appropriate measures (e.g. scoops, cans, bowls) are more reliable and faster to use. However, scales should be used periodically to check that volume measurements are accurate. As a rule, people should bring their own receptacles to collect their rations, but a reserve stock of empty bags, tins, and other containers should be kept for people who have nothing. Bottles for oil and tins to hold cereals and other commodities are usually easy to find.

Casual checks at local markets may indicate that beneficiaries have sold some of their rations or traded them for other foods. This is unavoidable and may even be appropriate when rations are qualitatively inadequate. Bulk sales, however, may reflect gross mismanagement by food relief personnel.

Ration cards

Care must be taken to ensure that each family (or household) receives only one card, which shows the number of individual rations to which it is entitled. This may be achieved by issuing cards on a house-to-house basis or at a meeting attended by the entire group. For displaced populations, cards may be distributed at the time of their first entry to a camp, for example. A typical ration card is shown in Fig. 9. The card should specify: the address; the name of head of family/household and home town/village; the total number of household members. It can be used to record the rations, blankets, and other items received. A stamp or some other form of official mark should be included on the card to avoid replication, forgery, or other abuses.

Fig. 9 Example of a household ration card

United Nations
High Commisioner
for Refugees

No. ET 0000000
Shelter No:

Date:

Clerk:

Name of Head of Family:

Persons: M F

Child: <6

Total:

Vulnerable: SP UM SF PD UE

Health Screening Comments

1	2	3	4	5
6	7	8	9	10

1 2 3 4 5 6 7 8 9 10 11 12 13 14 15 16 17 18 19 20 21 22 23 24 25 26 27 28 29 30

WHO 99260

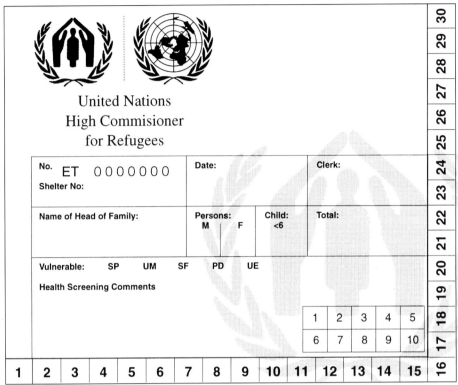

Key: Numbers 1–30: number of distributions (card is replaced after 30 distributions)
Numbers 1–10: number of individuals in family
SP: single parent
UM: unaccompanied minor
SF: single-female-headed household
PD: physically disabled
UE: unaccompanied elderly

Changes in the composition and size of individual families — including births, deaths, reunifications, or departures (e.g. for repatriation) — should be recorded as and when they occur, and procedures established for issuing new cards to eligible beneficiaries when necessary. Separate provision should be made for new arrivals, pending their formal registration and incorporation into the distribution system. Claims of lost cards are inevitable; some will be made by individuals attempting to obtain additional cards, but many will be genuine.

The loss of cards, the issue of new ones, and sometimes the volume of new arrivals will make it necessary periodically to conduct an exercise to reissue new cards to the entire population.

Authority to issue ration cards must be strictly controlled. All ration cards should be marked with a stamp that cannot be forged and is kept by the supervisor.

Fig. 10 Plan for distribution of dry food rations

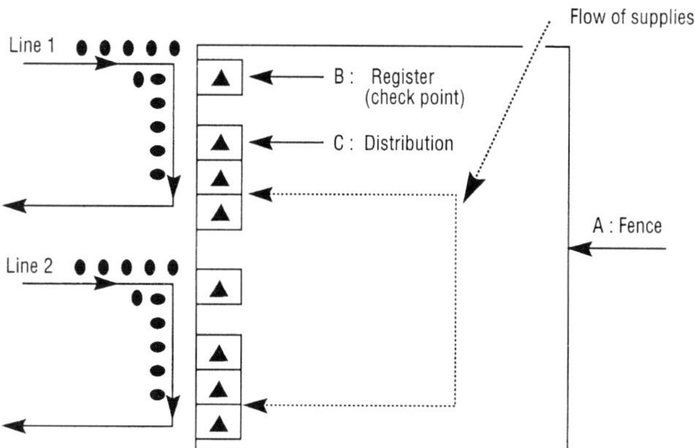

Key:
A Fence of mats, bamboo, wire, or rope, depending on needs and resources. Narrowing aisles for line-ups may also be necessary.
B Check-point for ration cards, sheltered by roof (or umbrella). The quantity of rations to be supplied should be called out clearly to distributors at C.
C Distribution point. Several bags at a time can be emptied onto a tarpaulin to speed up distribution.

General ration distributions in camp situations

The distribution area should be located near the store and fenced off. People should be directed to form several lines, which can be served simultaneously, and there should be a ration card check-point for each line (see Fig. 10). If the camp has 10 sectors, sectors 1 and 2 can receive rations on Monday, 3 and 4 on Tuesday, and so on. In a camp that is twice as large, rations can be distributed to sectors 1–5 one week and to sectors 6–10 the next.

Each distribution line will require a trained person to check cards, a person to distribute each commodity, and at least two people to control the crowd. Rubber stamps, containers for food, and standard measures for each commodity will be needed for each line.

At distribution time, heads of household (or family representatives) should line up and wait to be called. If the ground is dry, they can sit in line, which will prevent pushing and is much less tiring than standing for long periods, especially in the sun. In extreme climates, it may be necessary to provide shelter, and it is always essential to ensure that drinking-water is available in adequate quantities. Further details may be found in *Commodity distribution: a practical guide*.[1]

General ration distributions in villages

In villages, the elders or other local authorities can distribute relief supplies in fenced-off areas away from the market place or village centre. Rations should be distributed to family units/households on the basis of village registers or other

[1] *Commodity distribution: a practical guide*. Geneva, Office of the United Nations High Commissioner for Refugees, 1997.

official records of the village population. A simple list will suffice; individual ration cards are not necessary. However, the following are essential features of village distribution:

- *People should always be informed, well in advance, of the day on which food distribution will take place.* Regular distribution on fixed days is essential. It ensures that people will attend and will "budget" consumption between distributions.
- *Recipients must be aware of the amounts to which they are entitled.* Standard measures for cereals and other items should be publicly demonstrated. This reassures people that there is no cheating. It is also a good idea to carry out occasional re-weighing surveys of the food that people carry away from distribution points.

A group of villages may be served by a central store. Depending on the distances involved and the transport facilities available, village representatives can travel to the store on set days to collect the rations. Over short distances animals may be used to transport food. When plans are disrupted by the weather or by transport delays, people should be informed of this in good time.

The general administrative pattern for large-scale distribution, to whole regions or countries for example, is discussed in Chapter 7. At the local level, village authorities are usually responsible to the ministry of local government (or equivalent) at the district level. However, other government departments, such as the social services ministry, may be responsible for handling the food distribution down to the grassroots level. In any case there should be an intersectoral committee or subcommittee at the district level responsible for allocating rations and managing their distribution on an equitable basis in the affected communities. More details are given in Chapter 7.

Distributions among populations

No easy way has been found to distribute food to pastoral (nomadic) populations. Locations where people congregate, such as water sources, may be practical points from which to organize food distribution. Where regular contact with a pastoral population is difficult it may be sensible to give out larger amounts of food — up to 100 kg — at each distribution.

Large-scale cooked food distribution

Large-scale distribution of cooked food should be avoided except as a short-term measure that stops as soon as people have the necessary resources to prepare their own meals. The reasons for this are the following:

- Such programmes are often culturally inappropriate and may cause offence.
- Hygiene is difficult to ensure.
- Experience has shown that food intakes are often lower than intended: incorrect amounts of food are allocated when relief workers are confused by differences between weights or volumes of dry and cooked food.

- It is difficult to meet the needs of young children for frequent small meals or snacks. (Small children are unable to consume their whole daily requirement in two or even three meals.)

Types and quantities of cooked food for distribution

Cooked food should be the same as or similar to the normal diet. Whenever possible, local foods should be used. If non-traditional items have to be used, they should be prepared in a form as close as possible to local foods (soups, tortillas, chapatis, etc.). Spices are usually easy to obtain, are required in small quantities, and increase the acceptability of the food.

The quantity to be served should be calculated in terms of dry rations first (see Tables 21 and A2.1) and then as servings or meals per day. Many foods (especially cereals and pulses) increase substantially in volume during cooking; some double in volume while others, like rice, swell to four or five times the original volume.

Children need three or more meals a day, whereas two daily meals are probably sufficient for most adults.

Facilities for cooked food distribution

Kitchens should be sheltered, preferably inside buildings, and the surrounding area should be fenced off. As much space as possible should be set aside for the purpose. Space is needed for: storing water (a minimum of 10 litres per person per day); washing and cleaning food; initial preparation; cooking; briefly keeping prepared foods ready for service; and washing up. In a large camp, one kitchen should be set up for every 200–300 families (or 1000–1500 people).

Hygiene and food storage

Outbreaks of foodborne diseases are frequent in mass feeding situations. To prevent such outbreaks a number of basic rules should be observed:

- All kitchen supervisors, cooks, and ancillary personnel should be trained in personal hygiene and the principles of safe food preparation.[1]
- Cleaners should be employed to keep the kitchen and surrounding areas clean; they should be properly trained and their work supervised.
- Water and soap must be provided for personal cleanliness and detergent for cleaning utensils; there must be adequate facilities for waste disposal.
- Cooked food must not be stored, especially if it contains animal products.

Some types of local staple food, e.g. bread, can be kept in an edible condition for several days. Cold-mixed foods, e.g. milks, should be made up freshly before use with potable (boiled and cooled) water. They should never be kept standing in an uncovered container for more than a few minutes.

---

[1] For further guidelines on safe food preparation, see Annex 5 and *Health surveillance and management procedures for food-handling personnel. Report of a WHO consultation* (Geneva, World Health Organization, 1989; WHO Technical Report Series, No. 785).

Personnel and equipment

Any kitchen that distributes cooked foods requires cooks, cooks' assistants (to clean vegetables, make fires, carry water, etc.), cleaners, and people to wash up. Their number depends on the type and amount of food to be prepared. Camp residents should be employed whenever possible (see Chapter 7).

If foods are being cooked in bulk, large receptacles will be needed. On the other hand, preparation of large amounts of staple foods in individual portions requires a larger number of smaller utensils and more personnel. It may be necessary to obtain appropriate local cooking equipment.

When the food is to be prepared in individual portions, the number of portions that can be prepared in one hour should be determined by timing the preparation of 10 portions by a local cook. The number of cooks and cooking points required can then be calculated, as in the following example:

number of beneficiaries = 1000

number of meals per day = 3

number of portions required daily = 1000 × 3 = 3000

number prepared by one cook in one hour = 100

number of cook-hours required = 3000/100 = 30

time available for preparation = 6 hours

number of cooking points required = 30/6 = 5

number of cooks required = 5 + 2 (for rest periods) = 7

Each cooking point must be equipped with a full set of utensils.

For bulk preparation, requiring very large cooking pots, it is possible to use cut-down 200-litre petrol drums (see Fig. 11). Requirements are calculated as in the following example:

quantity of dry food per person per meal = 100 g

volume of one portion when cooked = 350–450 ml = 0.35–0.45 litre

number of people to be fed at one meal = 1000

total volume to be prepared for each meal = 0.35–0.45 × 1000 = 350–450 litres

(assuming that the food must be freshly prepared for each meal).

In practice, this means that at least four or five 100-litre cooking pots and two or three cooks would be required.

Additional utensils are required for:

- cooking soup (calculated as for staple prepared in bulk)
- mixing, soaking, or cleaning ingredients prior to cooking or fermentation (e.g. cereals, cassava, beans) where required
- mixing and serving the final meals.

Fig. 11 Using an oil drum as a cooking pot

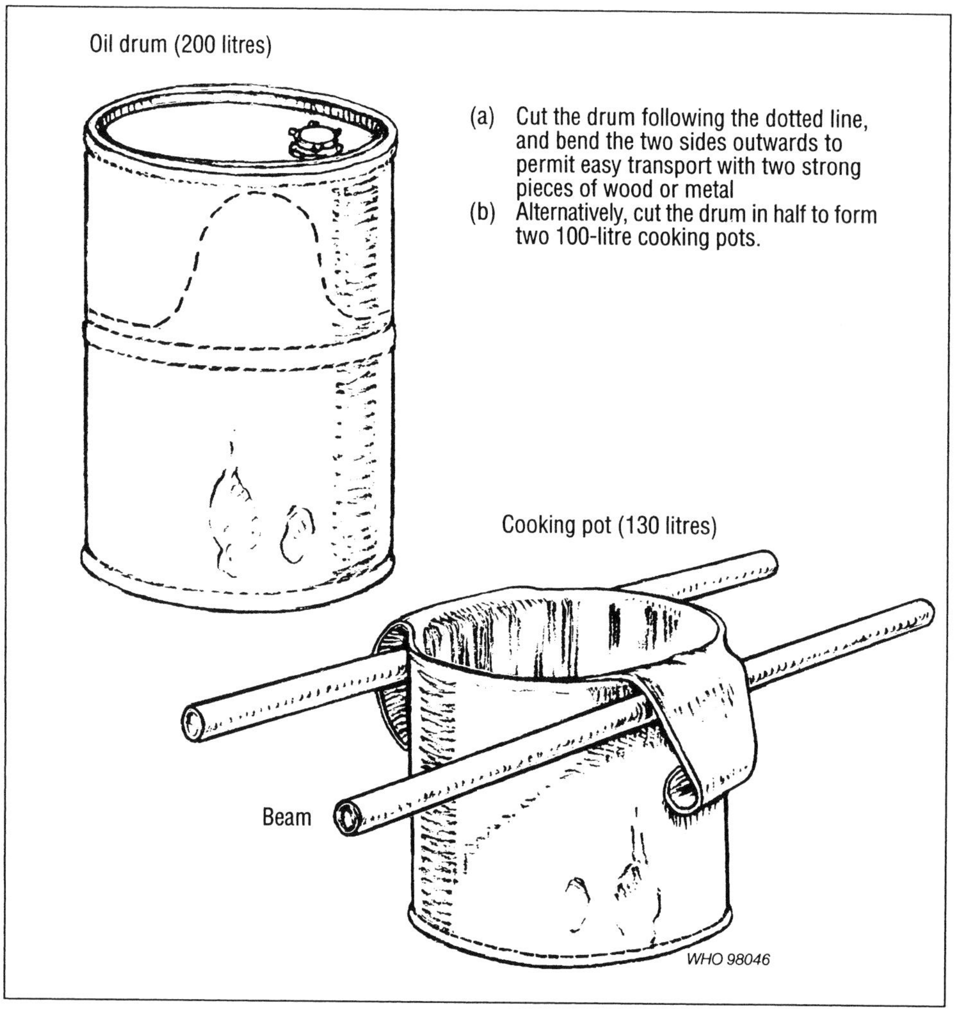

Oil drum (200 litres)

(a) Cut the drum following the dotted line, and bend the two sides outwards to permit easy transport with two strong pieces of wood or metal
(b) Alternatively, cut the drum in half to form two 100-litre cooking pots.

Cooking pot (130 litres)

Beam

WHO 98046

Cooking fuel

If wood, cow dung, or other local fuel is used, it is usually best to adopt the local method of building fires as well. To avoid having to collect fuel, each person or family receiving food may be asked to bring one piece of wood (or other fuel) to each meal. If local fuel collection is difficult or may cause deforestation, kerosene should be considered as an alternative.

Organization of distribution

Families who are to receive cooked rations should be registered and issued with ration cards in a manner similar to registration for dry ration distribution. At meal times, a representative of each household presents a card indicating the number of people to be fed. The combined ration is measured into a suitable container and the card is marked to indicate that the ration has been allocated.

In a large community or camp where there are several kitchens and distribution centres, it is important that recipients know which kitchen they are supposed to attend. The feeding supervisor should keep a register of all those to be fed from his or her kitchen.

Monitoring the effectiveness of a feeding programme

The effectiveness of each programme must be reviewed at regular intervals. The quantities of food distributed or the reported number of beneficiaries are *not*, in themselves, adequate measures. See Annex 7.

CHAPTER 5

Nutritional relief: selective feeding programmes

Selective feeding programmes provides additional food to specific vulnerable groups and those needing nutritional rehabilitation. It embraces two sub-categories — supplementary and therapeutic feeding programmes.

Supplementary feeding programmes may be needed when childhood malnutrition is very prevalent or is at risk of becoming prevalent. It provides additional food to nutritionally vulnerable groups, including moderately malnourished children and pregnant or lactating women, either through on-site feeding with cooked meals (500–700 $kcal_{th}$ per day) or by distribution of a dry take-home ration (1000–1200 $kcal_{th}$ per day). Breast-feeding must be encouraged, and wet nurses found if possible for infants who cannot be fed by their own mothers.

A supplementary feeding programme is only a safety net. Its general objective is to reduce the prevalence of malnutrition and mortality among vulnerable groups. It is *not* designed to "compensate" on a long-term basis for a general ration that is inadequate and should be improved.

Blanket supplementary feeding programmes should be needed only temporarily when malnutrition rates (weight-for-height below median −2 SD) exceed 15%, or 10% in the presence of other aggravating factors.

Targeted supplementary feeding (i.e. extra food given to selected individuals) is indicated if the malnutrition rate exceeds 10%, or 5% in the presence of other aggravating factors (e.g. high mortality and/or epidemic infectious diseases).

Therapeutic feeding is required to reduce the death rate among infants and young children suffering from severe protein–energy malnutrition. A rehabilitative diet, with high-energy foods served at frequent intervals, provides 150–200 $kcal_{th}$ and 2–3 g of protein per kg of body weight daily. For the first few days there must be close medical supervision and feeding every 3 hours on a 24-hour basis. Mothers should feed their sick children themselves.

Death often occurs in the first four days. The cause is usually infection and dehydration, which should be treated promptly; broad-spectrum antibiotics are very often needed, as is oral (or nasogastric) rehydration. Immunization against measles is a priority, and all severely malnourished children should receive normal doses of vitamin A.

Signs of recovery are: oedema loss, weight gain, and improvement of general condition. Failure to recover is mainly due to inadequate or faulty feeding or infections, including tuberculosis or HIV.

Introduction

The objective of a selective feeding programme is to reduce the prevalence of malnutrition and mortality among vulnerable groups. It must be very clear that selective feeding is not designed to compensate for the inadequacy of a general ration. Rather, the aim must be to improve general rations, if they are inadequate. A "decision tree" for the implementation of selective feeding programmes is shown in Fig. 12.

This chapter deals with selective feeding programmes of two types — supplementary and therapeutic feeding. Guiding principles for feeding infants and young children generally in emergency situations may be found in Annex 6.

Supplementary feeding

When there are significant levels of malnutrition and/or the general ration is not adequate, one possible course of action is to establish a supplementary feeding

Fig. 12 Decision chart for the implementation of selective feeding programmes

Note: This chart is for guidance only and should be adapted to local circumstances.

Finding		Action required
Food availablility at household level below 2100 $kcal_{th}$ per person per day	⇨	*Unsatisfactory situation:* • Improve general rations until local food availability and access can be made adequate
Malnutrition rate[a] 15% or more *or* 10–14% with aggravating factors[b]	⇨	*Serious situation:* • General rations (unless situation is limited to vulnerable groups); *plus* • Supplementary feeding generalized for all members of vulnerable groups, especially children and pregnant and lactating women • Therapeutic feeding programme for severely malnourished individuals
Malnutrition rate[a] 10–14% *or* 5–9% with aggravating factors[b]	⇨	*Risky situation* • No general rations; *but* • Supplementary feeding targeted to individuals identified as malnourished in vulnerable groups • Therapeutic feeding programme for severely malnourished individuals
Malnutrition rate[a] under 10% with no aggravating factors	⇨	*Acceptable situation:* • No need for population interventions • Attention for malnourished individuals through regular community services

[a] Malnutrition rate is defined as the percentage of the child population (6 months to 5 years) who are below either the reference median weight-for-height −2 SD or 80% of reference weight-for height.

[b] Aggravating factors:

— general food ration below the mean energy requirement

— crude mortality rate more than 1 per 10 000 per day

— epidemic of measles or whooping cough (pertussis)

— high incidence of respiratory or diarrhoeal diseases.

programme to protect vulnerable groups. This decision should be made locally by experienced personnel, and any programme should be planned and organized in close coordination with maternal and child health services.

Supplementary feeding is intended to supplement energy and/or nutrients missing from the basic diet of individuals who have special nutritional requirements or who are moderately malnourished. It is not necessary for a population that is adequately nourished and receiving a regular and suitable general ration. Vulnerable groups include moderately malnourished children, adolescents, malnourished pregnant and lactating women, individuals with chronic medical problems (e.g. tuberculosis), and the elderly.

Supplementary feeding programmes may consist of "take-home" dry rations for each registered individual, or "on-site" feedings of all registered persons with cooked meals. Infants who are not breast-fed are particularly prone to infection and malnutrition and should be watched closely; infant foods should never be prepared in advance and left at room temperature.

When to start a supplementary feeding programme

The decision to start a supplementary feeding programme (SFP) will be based on the following considerations:

- results of a nutrition survey — prevalence of acute malnutrition (using weight-for-height as indicator);
- the general food ration/food availability;
- child mortality rates and prevalence of specific diseases such as measles and whooping cough (pertussis);
- available resources (personnel, food) and logistic factors.

If a random anthropometric survey among children aged 6 months to 5 years points to more than 10% of them having weight-for-height values more than 2 SD below the reference median, a temporary supplementary and/or therapeutic feeding programme is justified. However, resources are always limited, and health workers should be careful not to allow a supplementary feeding centre to divert attention from the main problems in the population — insufficient or poor-quality general food rations or ineffective health services.

Two main types of SFP can be distinguished. The most common is the *targeted* supplementary feeding programme, which aims at the rehabilitation of malnourished children, adolescents, adults, and elderly people. It concentrates on the malnourished individuals, and should be implemented when the overall malnutrition rate among under-5s (more than 2 SD below the reference median) is 10–15%. A *blanket* supplementary feeding programme provides a food supplement for *all* children of a certain age, usually under 5 years,[1] plus pregnant women from the time of confirmed pregnancy (usually between 4 and 6 months) and lactating women until 6 months after delivery, in order to prevent an increase in the number who are malnourished. A blanket SFP is started when 15% or more

[1] In the case of infants under 6 months who are malnourished but breast-fed, the supplement should be given to the breast-feeding mothers, not to the infants.

of children are malnourished provided that sufficient resources (food, personnel) are available.

Blanket supplementary feeding programme

The principal characteristics of a blanket SFP may be summarized as follows:

Objectives:	prevent increase in PEM and micronutrient deficiency rates reduce excess mortality
Target group:	all children under 5 years of age and all individuals of other vulnerable groups, pregnant women from the time of confirmed pregnancy (usually between 4 and 6 months), and lactating women until 6 months after delivery
Features:	no individual monitoring or registration selection of children — less than 110 cm in length preventive medication — vitamin A, measles vaccination

Targeted supplementary feeding programme

The principal characteristics of a targeted SFP may be summarized as follows:

Objectives:	reduce prevalence of acute and severe malnutrition reduce excess mortality
Target group:	(see below)
Features:	individual registration, monitoring of weight, individual medical treatment

Target groups for targeted supplementary feeding programmes

A targeted SFP will target the following groups (in order of priority):

- malnourished children under 5 years (below 80% of reference median weight-for-height or more than 2 SD below reference median weight-for-height)
- malnourished individuals above 5 years of age

(both including those discharged from therapeutic feeding programmes)

- selected pregnant women and lactating mothers (until 6 months after delivery)
- individuals with social and medical problems (twins, orphans, unaccompanied children, the disabled, HIV-positive individuals, and tuberculosis patients)
- elderly people.

Based on a nutrition survey, the target population of a targeted SFP can be estimated as follows:

total population ×15% = population aged 6 months up to 5 years

(population aged 6 months up to 5 years) × malnutrition rate = total number of malnourished children to be reached

Example

Total camp population	50 000
Population aged 6 months up to 5 years (15%)	7500
Malnutrition rate	20%
Number of acutely malnourished children	= 7500 × 20% = **1500**

Adults are assessed for oedema and BMI as described in Chapter 3. Interpretation of results, however, will depend on circumstances. For instance, if a population is generally thin (in many countries the average BMI is around 18.5), only those individuals with BMI below, say, 17 (moderate thinness) would be considered to qualify for targeted feeding. On the other hand, if the population normally has a BMI value of 20 or above, 18.5 (marginal thinness) may be taken as a cut-off for targeted feeding. A BMI below 16 (severe thinness) is taken as clear indication of need for therapeutic feeding. BMI is not usually measured after the first trimester of pregnancy. There is a trend to supplement all pregnant women in emergency situations (or to select for supplementation on medical grounds). Flexibility and sound clinical judgment, both locally and within a national policy, are essential in determining the levels at which targeted and therapeutic feeding are considered, particularly as regards pregnant women. The decision may also be significantly influenced by the availability of foods.

How to start screening and selection

Once a nutrition survey (based on weight-for-height) has justified the implementation of a targeted SFP, the quickest way to identify all children who should be targeted is by means of population screening for mid-upper arm circumference (MUAC) and then weight-for-height, as described in Chapter 3. This may be summarized as follows:

- Screen all children aged 6–59 months (or height >65 cm, <110 cm) in the population, using MUAC.
- Further examine all children found to have MUAC below median −2 SD of MUAC for age or height.
- Select for supplementary feeding those children whose weight-for-height is between 2 and 3 SD below the median reference value, or between 70% and 80% of median reference value.
- Select for therapeutic feeding those children with weight-for-height more than 3 SD below, or less than 70% of, median reference value.

MUAC is a suitable tool for initial screening, but admission to the feeding programme will be based primarily on weight-for-height; however, the presence of oedema or an MUAC value for age or height below median −3 SD is an indicator of severe malnutrition, and justifies immediate admission to therapeutic feeding programmes.

In a settled population all households should be requested to bring children under 5 years or <110 cm to the feeding centre or child health clinic for screening. If this is not effective, children should be identified through home-visiting. Cooperation from the community is therefore essential for the programme. New arrivals in a refugee camp should be screened during registration.

Criteria for admission and discharge

In an emergency situation clearly defined anthropometric and illness criteria or cut-offs are needed for admission to and discharge from a selective feeding programme. The criteria and cut-off points selected should be in agreement with national relief policies.

Admission criteria

Admission criteria for selective feeding depend both on the objectives of the programme and on available resources. If resources are uncertain, more restrictive admission criteria should be applied; they can be altered during a programme according to specific circumstances such as a change in national policy or in available resources. The criteria will be based on age, nutritional status, and health status.

Age

- <59 months, or, if age is unknown, length <110 cm.
- Moderately or severely malnourished children older than 5 years.
- For malnourished infants under 6 months, it is the mothers who should be included in the programme, *not* the infants (who should be exclusively breast-fed).

  The nutritional status of young infants depends to some extent on the nutritional status of their mothers (except for children at special risk, such as orphans or twins). When a mother is severely malnourished or suffering from severe infection or overwork, she may produce inadequate breast milk, leading to malnutrition of the infant. Breast-milk production may also be affected by psychosocial factors. Hence an additional supplementary ration for the mother may be advisable (particularly if the general ration is not totally adequate), as well as proper health care.

Nutritional status

- *Moderate malnutrition.* Weight-for-height between 2 and 3 SD below median reference value (or between 70 and 80% of median reference value).
- *Severe malnutrition.* Children more than 3 SD below the reference value or less than 70% of the reference value and/or with oedema in both feet. All children with these signs should immediately be referred to a therapeutic feeding centre or to a hospital if possible.

Health status

- Children who are moderately underweight (between 2 and 3 SD below median weight-for-length or 70–80% of median) but severely ill, e.g. with associated measles, pneumonia, or diarrhoeal disease, should be considered for therapeutic feeding.
- Children undergoing rehabilitation, i.e. recovering from severe malnutrition, for which they have received therapeutic feeding, and ready for discharge

from the therapeutic feeding programme (see page 93), should receive supplementary feeding for at least 3 months to prevent relapse, which is otherwise extremely common.

Discharge criteria

Criteria for discharging children from a targeted SFP are as follows:

- Usually, attainment of weight-for-height 1.5 SD below the reference median, or 85% of reference median, maintained for two consecutive weighings one week apart.
- If resources are limited, discharge may be based simply on attainment of weight-for-height 2 SD below the reference median or 80% of the reference median on two consecutive measurements.

A targeted SFP should continue as long as prevalence of malnutrition is still 15% or more.

Type of feeding programme: wet or dry

Supplementary feeding intended for moderately malnourished individuals can take two forms: wet or dry. Wet feeding relies on 1–4 prepared meals daily consumed "on-site". Malnourished children have to be brought to the feeding centre every day by parents or caregivers. In a "dry" feeding programme, dry rations are distributed (usually weekly) to be taken home for preparation and consumption.

There are advantages and disadvantages to both types of ration, but no clear evidence as to which type of feeding programme is more effective for combating malnutrition. Because resources (staff, materials) are limited in many emergency situations, the possibility of a dry feeding programme should always be considered first; it may even be the only feasible option. Some advantages of dry feeding are:

- it is easier to organize than a wet feeding programme when resources (staff, materials) are limited;
- it can serve more children than a wet feeding programme;
- it poses a lower risk than a wet feeding programme of transmission of communicable diseases among highly vulnerable malnourished children;
- it takes up less of the mothers' limited time;
- it achieves better coverage of children under 2 years than a wet feeding programme;
- it is more easily accessible for a dispersed population;
- in famine situations in which people are still in their own homes, it helps to prevent their displacement.

A wet feeding programme has advantages in situations where:

- cooking facilities (fuel, pots) are a major problem in the community;

- security is poor, e.g. when it is feared that women carrying their dry rations home will be robbed along the way.

When to close down a supplementary feeding programme

A supplementary feeding programme can be closed down when the number of malnourished children is reduced, so that fewer than 10% of the children under 5 years are malnourished. This must be verified by a nutritional survey. It may then become more effective to manage individual malnourished cases through other health facilities. However, the following conditions should be met before the programme is closed:

- general food distributions are reliable and adequate;
- public health and disease control measures are effective;
- no seasonal deterioration of nutritional status is expected;
- mortality among children under 5 years is low;
- no major population influx is expected.

There must be follow-up nutrition surveys (preferably 3-monthly) and regular food-basket monitoring in order to detect any deterioration of conditions, especially if the overall situation remains unstable.

Foods and rations for supplementary feeding

The supplementary food should provide 500–700 $kcal_{th}$ per beneficiary per day and should include 15–25 g of protein. The majority of those registered for supplementary feeding will usually be small children. To ensure that the food is eaten, it must be palatable and rich in energy and nutrients, but low in bulk. A 1-year-old can usually consume a maximum of 300 ml at a meal. This implies that a porridge used for feeding should provide at least 1 $kcal_{th}$/ml.

Supplementary rations for refugees and other large populations affected by emergencies are often based partially or largely on specially-blended cereal mixtures such as corn–soy blend (CSB), with oil and/or sugar. Where dried skim milk (DSM) is available and hygienic preparation can be assured, DSM/oil/sugar mixes are sometimes used. Although these foods are convenient to use, they are not essential. Commodities available in the general ration — including cereals, pulses, and oil — can be used to make satisfactory supplementary rations and are cheaper.

Table 22 provides examples of rations for supplementary feeding based on the imported food aid commodities that have been used in many assistance operations for refugees and displaced persons. **The quantities indicated are for on-site feeding. For take-home food distributions, quantities should be increased and the commodities should be distributed in the form of a pre-mix.** Where feasible, food for on-site supplementary feeding should be prepared in the form of traditional meals reinforced, where necessary, with additional quantities of oil and some fortified cereal blend.

Cereal blends or processed cereals can be prepared in ways similar to traditional foods. Some methods of preparation are given in Annex 5. Most blended foods

Table 22 Examples of rations for supplementary feeding

Commodity	Ration 1 (g)	Ration 2 (g)	Ration 3 (g)
On-site supplementary feeding[a]			
Blended food, fortified	100	—	—
Cereal (e.g. maize flour)	—	125	60
DSM	—	—	45
Pulses	—	30	—
Oil	30	20	30
Sugar	20	—	15
Salt	—	5	—
Energy ($kcal_{th}$)	725	700	700
Protein (% of energy)	10	11	12.5
Commodity	**Ration 1 (g)**	**Ration 2[b] (g)**	**Ration 3 (g)**
Take-home supplementary feeding[c]			
Blended food, fortified	200	140	250
DSM	—	50	—
Oil	20	50	25
Sugar	15	30	20
Energy ($kcal_{th}$)	1000	1250	1250
Protein (% of energy)	14	14.5	14.5

[a] On-site (wet) rations should normally supply (per ration):
energy: 500–700 $kcal_{th}$.
protein: 10–12% of energy.

[b] The commodities in this ration should be distributed as a pre-mix.

[c] Take-home (dry) rations should normally supply (per ration):
energy: 1000–1200 $kcal_{th}$.
protein: 10–12% of energy.

are precooked and have the advantage of being quickly prepared with cold water,[1] but care must be taken to avoid their contamination during reconstitution.

High-energy biscuits are sometimes used for supplementary feeding programmes, especially when cereal/pulse blends cannot be used.

Selection of beneficiaries

Beneficiaries may include those categories of individuals listed on page 77.[2]

Supplementary feeding centres

Supplementary feeding centres should be located within walking distance for small children. In a large camp several small centres are better than one large centre; small centres are more easily managed, the environment is pleasanter for mothers and children, and record-keeping for individual children is simpler.

Ration cards and attendance records

Ration cards for supplementary feeding are issued to the selected individuals. If possible, however, cards should not be given to children as they are easily dam-

[1] Cooking is advisable, however, for children under 3 years old.

[2] Criteria and methods for screening (selecting) children are described in Chapter 3.

aged or lost (or exchanged between children). Instead, plastic identity bracelets, metal tags, pieces of cloth or other resistant material, marked with a number, should be given to the mothers or carers. In "on-site" supplementary feeding programmes, the object of issuing ration cards or other identification is not to prevent children from being served twice but to provide a record of attendance. Health screening is also easier when children come regularly to supplementary feeding centres.

In a "take-home" system, ration cards (or other identification) are also necessary, not only to provide a record of attendance but also to ensure that only one ration is given out for each selected beneficiary.

At the centre, the attendance of individual children should be recorded in a register and/or on the individual cards. Children should be weighed monthly to assess their progress. Records are also used to:

- follow up children who do not attend regularly
- estimate the coverage of the supplementary feeding programme — if estimates of the numbers of potentially eligible beneficiaries are available from surveys, feeding centre records may be used to calculate the approximate proportion of those children who actually attend the centres.

Complementary public health interventions

Infections can contribute significantly to a deterioration in nutritional status. Even when the incidence and prevalence of an infection do not yet constitute a public health problem, the conditions that are common in emergencies (e.g. overcrowding, unsafe water supplies, poor sanitation, undernutrition, irregular health services) can be conducive to rapid and even disastrous spread, both locally (e.g. within a camp) and on a much larger scale. Adequate curative and preventive measures and health promotion activities should be integral to the management of a nutritional emergency.

Therapeutic feeding of children

An effective therapeutic feeding programme can significantly reduce mortality rates in a severely malnourished population. Effective therapeutic feeding requires well trained personnel and professional supervision, plus adequate resources (feeding materials, pharmaceuticals, water, utensils, etc.). In the early stages of an emergency, none of these may be available in sufficient quantity. However, therapeutic feeding should be started immediately, with whatever resources are available, in any situation where there are large numbers of severely malnourished children. This topic is treated in more detail in another WHO publication.[1]

---

[1] *Management of severe malnutrition: a manual for physicians and other senior health workers.* Geneva, World Health Organization, 1999.

Therapeutic feeding centres

Ideally, therapeutic feeding centres for severely malnourished children should be residential and serve no more than 50 children at a time. Whether they meet these ideal conditions or not, therapeutic feeding centres should provide *at least 6–8 meals daily*, of which at least one should be given in the middle of the night.

Each child should have an attendant — the mother, if possible. Mothers or other carers (not official personnel) will be responsible for the children's care and feeding and should be allowed to bring along their other children if it facilitates their participation.

Sometimes security problems or cultural constraints make it impossible to conduct therapeutic feeding on an inpatient (residential) basis. One option then is to set up day-care centres that provide 6–8 meals a day on an outpatient basis, and provide mothers with uncooked food[1] to give to children at night. Outpatient therapeutic feeding services can be quite effective, but are rarely successful in treating the most severe cases of PEM. Nevertheless, attendance of a child as an inpatient, or even as a daily outpatient, may well place a tremendous physical and economic burden on the mother. If she is normally in employment, or working in the fields, the rest of the family may depend on her for daily subsistence. Her being at the feeding centre full-time or for a large part of each day may have disastrous consequences for the family. The benefits of the intensive care that can be provided should therefore be carefully weighed against the stresses incurred. In some circumstances, giving rations to the mother and explaining carefully how to use them for therapeutic feeding at home, with periodic supervision, may be just as successful as residential therapy. The rations should be issued daily if possible, or at least weekly, with clear initial instructions and practice in their preparation. The child's condition should be checked, if possible by a physician or nurse, at each visit, to assess progress or deterioration, and procedures, including feeding instructions, should be modified if necessary.

Clearly, careful organization and intensive supervision are just as important in "domestic" treatment as in a residential centre. Costs, however, can be very much lower, and this may be a crucial consideration where resources are severely constrained. Domestic therapeutic feeding can be quite widely established — even in large populations — with modest resources that would be totally inadequate for residential facilities.

Admission criteria

Children should be admitted to therapeutic feeding centres if they have:

- weight-for-height values more than 3 SD below the reference median or less than 70% of the reference median (marasmus); and/or
- oedema (kwashiorkor) or marasmic kwashiorkor.

The criteria can be modified in accordance with national guidelines, the resources of the centre, and the capacity for follow-up, but they should always be clearly defined.

---

[1] This can be a dry mixture of dried skim milk, sugar, and oil (with instructions on how to mix with boiled water) or a high-energy biscuit.

When facilities are very limited, the weight-for-height standard may be lowered to median −4 SD or to 65% or 60% of reference median. Uncomplicated cases can be treated at home if they can be seen daily.

General procedures for treatment of severe PEM

Three phases are recognized in the general management of severe PEM. These, and errors to be avoided, are discussed in the following paragraphs.

- *Initial treatment phase*

  The initial treatment phase begins with admission to the therapeutic feeding centre and lasts until the child's condition is stable and his or her appetite has returned (usually after 2–7 days).

  During the acute phase (1–2 days) the main concerns are treatment and prevention. Complications commonly include dehydration from diarrhoea and vomiting; localized and generalized infections; septic shock; hypothermia and hypoglycaemia; anaemia and vitamin A deficiency; and other metabolic disorders, such as disorders of fluid and electrolytes in the body, that may easily given rise to sudden death.

  Dehydration and its management are dealt with in more detail in Chapter 6. Infections in severely malnourished children are often difficult to detect; for instance, there may be no rise in temperature until recovery is well under way. Careful examination is therefore essential; untreated infections may prevent or delay recovery. It is wise to give a course of antimicrobials to all children with severe malnutrition. Septic shock has similar signs to dehydration and needs broad-spectrum antibiotic treatment. Abnormally low temperature and/or blood sugar are common causes of death. Children with these problems must be kept warm and fed frequently with a formula diet (every 2–4 hours, day and night) to avoid collapse. Management of anaemia and vitamin A deficiency is described in Chapter 2.

  It must be emphasized that **acute, severe PEM is as much a medical emergency as, say, a heart attack**. Even with the utmost care, mortality rates are often 20–30% or higher. Deaths commonly occur during the first 24–48 hours after admission, and constant nursing care during this period is highly desirable. The main concerns include:

  — Frequent feeding, preferably with small amounts at this stage, since larger intakes are associated with higher mortality; for this purpose food is usually given in the form of a formula diet (see Table 23), and often through a nasogastric tube (see Annex 6) if the child is too weak or has no appetite. The aim is to provide only the child's approximate maintenance requirements, i.e. 80–100 $kcal_{th}$ per kg of body weight per day. Details of feeding are given below.

  — To prevent the child becoming cold.

  — To prevent or treat hidden infections — appropriate antibiotic therapy is often advisable (see section on medical care, below).

  This precarious phase may last as much as a week. During this time oedema may be lost in subjects with kwashiorkor, whose body weight therefore de-

***Table 23** Composition of F-75 and F-100 diets*

Constituent	Amount per 100 ml	
	F-75	F-100
Energy	75 $kcal_{th}$	100 $kcal_{th}$
Protein	0.9 g	2.9 g
Lactose	1.3 g	4.2 g
Potassium	3.6 mmol	5.9 mmol
Sodium	0.6 mmol	1.9 mmol
Magnesium	0.43 mmol	0.73 mmol
Zinc	2.0 mg	2.3 mg
Copper	0.25 mg	0.25 mg
Percentage of energy from:		
protein	5%	12%
fat	32%	53%
Osmolarity	333 mOsmol/l	419 mOsmol/l

creases; this can be a favourable sign. Oedema itself is not a sign of particular danger, in that its presence does not make the outcome worse, nor does it call for the use of diuretics.

Very sick children need very frequent feeding with a formula diet containing less protein and more sugar (F-75 in Table 23). As soon as they can manage it, they should progress to the more concentrated F-100 liquid diet (see Table 23) which can be continued into the rehabilitation phase if resources permit.

- *Rehabilitation phase*

  The child is deemed to have entered the rehabilitation phase when his or her appetite has returned. However, at the start of the rehabilitation phase, the child is still deficient in protein and various micronutrients, including potassium, magnesium, iron, and zinc. These must be given in increased amounts. Infants under 24 months of age can be fed exclusively on liquid or semi-liquid formulas. It is usually appropriate to introduce solid foods for older children. The rate of recovery depends to a large extent on the daily intake. The child should be encouraged and stimulated by constant care, social contact, and play. As recovery proceeds, appetite eventually tends to decline again. Usually this phase lasts 2–6 weeks. There is no clear evidence of much advantage in a longer stay in a residential rehabilitation centre; if the child is eating well, food supplies are adequate, and good care is possible at home, rehabilitation can proceed satisfactorily at home with a weekly outpatient check.

From this brief overview it will be apparent that severe PEM is a medical emergency and its management is complex. Nevertheless, if parents can be properly instructed and motivated to feed children 4-hourly day and night, with small amounts at first, gradually increasing, children may in fact do as well at home as in the hospital environment where, in emergency situations, the available foods, personnel, and facilities are often less than optimal.

Errors to avoid in therapeutic feeding

A number of errors are to be avoided in therapeutic feeding. They are listed here, but more details are given in another WHO publication:[1]

- inappropriate or unnecessary use of drugs, especially for diarrhoea;
- superficial and infrequent examination of patients;
- unnecessary or contraindicated aggressive treatment;
- intravenous feeding;
- long intervals between feeds;
- lack of personnel and of time to feed patients and supervise their food intake;
- inadequate protection in cold environments;
- hasty or frequent changes of treatment without appropriate evaluation;
- lack of emotional and psychological stimulation;
- untrained cooks and unsafe handling of foods;
- frequent changes of staff;
- restrictions on involvement of mothers and other relatives;
- inadequate instruction to the child's parents (or carers);
- premature discharge without referral to another site to complete the recovery.

General procedures for therapeutic feeding

Each child should be weighed on admission, and daily thereafter. Weight gain is the main indicator of progress after the disappearance of oedema and after infections, dehydration, etc. have been controlled.

During the acute phase the child is very vulnerable and needs constant monitoring. The first priority is to restore normal blood sugar levels, body temperature, hydration, and electrolyte balance, and to treat infections — including septic shock — and any other problems. Feeding should start at this time. The very sick child can manage only easily digested liquid feeds and should be fed little and often.

If the child is dehydrated, a modified solution of oral rehydration salts (ORS) should be given. This can be made by dissolving one packet of the standard ORS in 2 litres of water (instead of 1 litre) and adding 50 g of sucrose and 40 ml of mineral mix solution (see Table 24).

In the acute phase, F-75 liquid formula should be given throughout the day and night, every 2–3 hours at first, then 4-hourly as the child starts to take more. Breast-feeding should continue. If the child is unwilling to take the formula, it can be given through a nasogastric tube (feeding little and often to avoid overloading the intestine, liver, and kidneys). The child should receive

[1] *Management of severe malnutrition: a manual for physicians and other senior health workers.* Geneva, World Health Organization, 1999.

Table 24 *Composition of mineral mix solution*

Constituent	Amount
Potassium chloride	89.5 g
Tripotassium citrate	32.4 g
Magnesium chloride ($MgCl_2 \cdot 6H_2O$)	30.5 g
Zinc acetate	3.3 g
Copper sulfate	0.56 g
Sodium selenate[a]	10 mg
Potassium iodide[a]	5 mg
Water to make	1000 ml

[a] If it is not possible to weigh very small amounts accurately, this substance may be omitted.

Table 25 *Volumes of F-75 diet to give at each feed to achieve a daily intake of 100 kcal$_{th}$/kg*

Weight of child (kg)	Volume of F-75 per feed (ml)[a]		
	Every 2 hours (12 feeds)	Every 3 hours (8 feeds)	Every 4 hours (6 feeds)
2.0	20	30	45
2.2	25	35	50
2.4	25	40	55
2.6	30	45	55
2.8	30	45	60
3.0	35	50	65
3.2	35	55	70
3.4	35	55	75
3.6	40	60	80
3.8	40	60	85
4.0	45	65	90
4.2	45	70	90
4.4	50	70	95
4.6	50	75	100
4.8	55	80	105
5.0	55	80	110
5.2	55	85	115
5.4	60	90	120
5.6	60	90	125
5.8	65	95	130
6.0	65	100	130
6.2	70	100	135
6.4	70	105	140
6.6	75	110	145
6.8	75	110	150
7.0	75	115	155
7.2	80	120	160
7.4	80	120	160
7.6	85	125	165
7.8	85	130	170
8.0	90	130	175
8.2	90	135	180
8.4	90	140	185
8.6	95	140	190
8.8	95	145	195
9.0	100	145	200
9.2	100	150	200
9.4	105	155	205
9.6	105	155	210
9.8	110	160	215
10.0	110	160	220

[a] Rounded to the nearest 5 ml.

80–100 $kcal_{th}$/kg of body weight per day. Table 25 indicates the volumes of F-75 feed to give.

The return of appetite usually occurs after 2–7 days and indicates that the child's condition has improved significantly. The rehabilitation phase now starts. The child's appetite and general condition, *not* the time elapsed since the start of treatment, should dictate when rehabilitation can start. At this stage the F-75 liquid formula can be gradually replaced by the F-100 formula. At first, the amounts should remain the same (to avoid heart failure resulting from a sudden increase in the volume of feed). After 2 days the quantities of F-100 formula can be increased (by 10 ml at each feed) until some food is left after most feeds. When the child is increasing in weight, feeding frequency can be reduced (to every 4 hours, day and night, i.e. six feeds per 24 hours) as the quantity of feed per meal increases. One night-time feed can be omitted when the child is growing well (making five feeds per 24 hours). The usual amount the child will accept is 150–220 $kcal_{th}$/kg of body weight per day. Any amount less than 130 $kcal_{th}$/kg per day is an indication that the child is failing to respond to treatment. The F-100 formula supplies 100 $kcal_{th}$/100 ml, so that the usual volume of F-100 formula accepted is between 150 and 220 ml/kg body weight per day, and the lowest acceptable intake is 130 ml/kg per day.

Children in the rehabilitation phase still need active encouragement to feed sufficiently. They should never be left alone to "take what they want". Breast-feeding should continue before, during, and after the rehabilitation phase.

The F-100 formula is also suitable for children over 24 months of age, but these children should also be introduced to solid food during rehabilitation when their appetites are restored. The supplementary food rations are suitable. It is important to ensure that the energy content is sufficient (which implies the use of oil) and that there are sufficient vitamins and minerals (often missing from the food available to the family). A suitable regime is to give F-100 three times daily and mixed diet three times daily — a total of six meals a day.

Before being discharged from the rehabilitation centre, the child and his or her mother or other care-giver should be prepared. The F-100 formula should be gradually withdrawn and the amount of mixed diet increased. The importance of frequent feeding with adequate amounts of a good mixed diet, including breast-feeding, needs to be explained to the mother or care-giver, who may need to be given extra rations for this purpose.

Preparation of feeding mixtures for therapeutic feeding

The F-75 and F-100 diets can easily be prepared from the basic ingredients — dried skim milk (DSM), sugar, cereal flour, oil, mineral mix, and vitamin mix (see Table 26). They are also commercially available as powder formulations that can be mixed with water.

The basic ingredients can be mixed together in bulk, and the resulting "pre-mix" stored in clean, covered containers for several days, depending on the local climate and the quality of the oil. Small quantities of the pre-mix can then be diluted with water as and when needed. Once mixed with water, the mixture must be used rapidly; liquid preparations must not be kept for more than 6 hours.

Table 26 *Preparation of F-75 and F-100 diets*

Ingredient	Amount	
	F-75[a–d]	F-100[e,f]
Dried skim milk	25 g	80 g
Sugar	70 g	50 g
Cereal flour	35 g	—
Vegetable oil	27 g	60 g
Mineral mix[g]	20 ml	20 ml
Vitamin mix[g]	140 mg	140 mg
Water to make	1000 ml	1000 ml

[a] To prepare the F-75 diet, add the dried skim milk, sugar, cereal flour, and oil to some water and mix. Boil for 5–7 minutes. Allow to cool, then add the mineral mix and vitamin mix and mix again. Make up the volume to 1000 ml with water.

[b] A comparable formula can be made from 35 g of whole dried milk, 70 g of sugar, 35 g of cereal flour, 17 g of oil, 20 ml of mineral mix, 140 mg of vitamin mix, and water to make 1000 ml. Alternatively, use 300 ml of fresh cow's milk, 70 g of sugar, 35 g of cereal flour, 17 g of oil, 20 ml of mineral mix, 140 mg of vitamin mix, and water to make 1000 ml.

[c] Isotonic versions of F-75 (280 mOsmol/l), which contain maltodextrins instead of cereal flour and some of the sugar and which include all the necessary micronutrients, are available commercially.

[d] If cereal flour is not available or there are no cooking facilities, a comparable formula can be made from 25 g of dried skim milk, 100 g of sugar, 27 g of oil, 20 ml of mineral mix, 140 mg of vitamin mix, and water to make 1000 ml. However, this formula has a high osmolarity (415 mOsmol/l) and may not be well tolerated by all children, especially those with diarrhoea.

[e] To prepare the F-100 diet, add the dried skim milk, sugar, and oil to some warm boiled water and mix. Add the mineral mix and vitamin mix and mix again. Make up the volume to 1000 ml with water.

[f] A comparable formula can be made from 110 g of whole dried milk, 50 g of sugar, 30 g of oil, 20 ml of mineral mix, 140 mg of vitamin mix, and water to make 1000 ml. Alternatively, use 880 ml of fresh cow's milk, 75 g of sugar, 20 g of oil, 20 ml of mineral mix, 140 mg of vitamin mix, and water to make 1000 ml.

[g] See Table 24 for mineral mix composition and Table 27 for vitamin mix. If only small amounts of feed are being prepared, it will not be feasible to prepare the vitamin mix because of the small amounts involved. In this case, give a proprietary multivitamin supplement. Alternatively, a combined mineral and vitamin mix for malnourished children is available commercially and can be used in the above diets.

Administering the food

Feeding sick children requires great patience. Mothers or other carers should be shown how to use the feeds for their children, but may need help and encouragement initially if the children have difficulty taking the food.

- A cup and/or spoon should be used for feeding.
- Initially, only liquid formula feeds should be given.
- After 2–7 days, semi-solid food can be introduced. Liquid formula feeds can be gradually replaced by a traditional diet, following the customs in the area, but this should be supplemented with extra energy (especially oil), adequate protein (by adding milk if necessary), vegetables, and fruits.
- For all infants and young children, breast-feeding should be continued in addition to solid feeding.
- Feeding should be continued, even if a child occasionally vomits.
- Any child with a communicable disease (e.g. confirmed tuberculosis or measles) should be kept and treated separately from others to avoid cross-infection. New admissions should be kept isolated from other residents for the first few days if possible.

Table 27 *Composition of vitamin mix*

Vitamin	Amount per litre of liquid diet
Water-soluble	
Thiamine (vitamin B_1)	0.7 mg
Riboflavin (vitamin B_2)	2.0 mg
Nicotinic acid	10 mg
Pyridoxine (vitamin B_6)	0.7 mg
Cyanocobalamin (vitamin B_{12})	1 μg
Folic acid	0.35 mg
Ascorbic acid (vitamin C)	100 mg
Pantothenic acid (vitamin B_5)	3 mg
Biotin	0.1 mg
Fat-soluble	
Retinol (vitamin A)	1.5 mg
Calciferol (vitamin D)	30 μg
α-Tocopherol (vitamin E)	22 mg
Vitamin K	40 μg

- If absolutely necessary, a nasogastric tube can be used for feeding during the first few days of treatment. Indications are: very poor appetite, weakness, painful stomatitis, vomiting, lack of cooperation by the mother, and failure to gain weight (in a non-oedematous child). However, feeding with a nasogastric tube is an emergency measure and should not be undertaken unless all else fails. Instructions on the use of nasogastric tubes are provided in Annex 6.

Medical care and medicines

Food is the specific therapy for PEM.

The following points may be helpful to those responsible for therapeutic feeding centres:

- *Drugs*. Other drugs should be given only when essential. Experience has shown that staff may waste considerable time giving unnecessary and expensive medicines instead of supervising intensive feeding.
- *Antimicrobials*. In extremely malnourished children infections may produce no fever or local signs; instead, they cause low blood sugar, hypothermia (rectal temperature <35.5 °C, underarm temperature <35 °C), apathy, and drowsiness. Bacteria normally found only in the large intestine often invade the small intestine. Death can easily result from this problem and/or from lower respiratory tract infections. The WHO manual on severe malnutrition[1] recommends that all children with severe malnutrition should routinely receive broad-spectrum antimicrobial treatment when first admitted for care. Doses should be based on a child's actual body weight; the dose of any drug normally given according to age should be *reduced in proportion to the child's deficit in body weight*, since overdose effects can easily occur in severely malnourished children. The recommended antimicrobials are:
  - co-trimoxazole (sulfamethoxazole 25 mg + trimethoprim 5 mg per kg) orally twice daily for 5 days;

[1] *Management of severe malnutrition: a manual for physicians and other senior health workers.* Geneva, World Health Organization, 1999.

— if there are complications, ampicillin, amoxicillin, and gentamicin, with added chloramphenicol if the child fails to improve in 48 hours.

- A measles outbreak in a feeding centre can be disastrous; all children over 6 months of age should be immunized against the disease on admission (see Chapter 6). A second dose of vaccine should be given before discharge.
- All children should receive a course of vitamin A therapy on admission (see Chapter 2 and Table 16).
- Anthelmintics can be administered routinely during the rehabilitation phase.
- It is also advisable to administer iron and folic acid (tablets or preferably liquid preparations) daily, but only after initiation of recovery. Children with moderate or severe anaemia should be given elemental iron, 3 mg/kg per day in two divided doses, up to a maximum of 60 mg daily for 3 months. All children must be given 5 mg of folic acid on day 1 then 1 mg/day thereafter.
- Multivitamin preparations are expensive and inefficient. It is better to prevent or treat specifically the mineral or vitamin deficiencies that are prevalent in the area.
- Modified oral rehydration solution should be available and administered to all severely malnourished children with diarrhoea.
- If a child does not respond to therapy and remains very ill, tuberculosis or AIDS should be suspected and treated appropriately.

Signs of recovery

Loss of oedema

Loss of oedema (in kwashiorkor) is an important sign of recovery. It usually happens after 5–9 days of therapeutic feeding. There is concomitant weight loss, as water is eliminated from the body. This phase is called "initiation of cure".

Weight gain

Children with PEM, including kwashiorkor patients after loss of oedema, should gain weight at a rate of 10–15 g per kg of body weight every day. A child who does not gain *at least* 5 g/kg per day for 3 consecutive days is failing to respond to treatment. The target weight is 1.5 SD below the median reference weight-for-length/height (see Table A3.1)

Improvement in general condition

A child's general condition is improving if appetite increases, behaviour is alert, and the stools are normal. It is important to monitor progress daily if possible, or at least every 2–3 days, and the child's weight should be recorded on a chart.[1] One chart should be kept for each child, and its meaning should be carefully explained to the mother or carer. It is helpful to record the target weight on the chart.

---

[1] Suitable charts may be found in: *Management of severe malnutrition: a manual for physicians and other senior health workers* (Geneva, World Health Organization, 1999).

Criteria for discharge

Before being discharged from a therapeutic feeding programme patients should have lost all oedema and weight-for-height should have reached at least −2SD or 80% of the NCHS/WHO median reference values on two consecutive weighings 1 week apart. They should be clinically examined before discharge and transfer to the supplementary feeding programme. They should also be active and free from infection.

Discharged children should be followed up on a regular basis, at least monthly, to minimize the risk of relapse. To reduce the possibility of relapse after discharge:

- a child should be enrolled for supplementary feeding and receive food supplements for at least 3 months (the aim is to reach the target weight);
- the mother or carer should understand how to feed the child correctly with the foods available.

Complications

Death typically occurs in 10–20% of children who have such severe PEM that they require therapeutic feeding, usually within the first 4 days after admission. Dehydration and septic shock are the major causes, but death may also be due to metabolic causes (hypoglycaemia, etc.), especially on the first or second night after admission.

It is essential to prevent, watch for, and respond promptly to the following problems:

- failure to gain weight
- hypothermia (rectal temperature below 35.5 °C (95.9 °F), underarm temperature below 35 °C (95.0 °F))
- severe anaemia
- lactose intolerance (intolerance to the sugar of non-human milks)
- hypoglycaemia (lack of sugar in the blood)
- infections.

Failure to gain weight

Most malnourished children who receive these special liquid formula feedings recover in 2–6 weeks. However, some fail to respond to treatment and to gain weight satisfactorily for the following reasons:

- a problem with feeding, such as incorrect preparation of food, unappetizing food, lack of persistence in feeding by the care-giver, or inadequate quantity or frequency of feeds; or
- a medical problem, such as an infection, worm infestation, amoebiasis, tuberculosis, or lactose intolerance.

If there is a failure to start to lose oedema by day 4 after admission and if oedema is still present on day 10, *or* if there is a failure to gain at least 5 g/kg of body weight by day 10 after admission, the child should be medically examined and may require more frequent or nasogastric feeding. In areas where tuberculosis is common, any malnourished child who does not gain weight satisfactorily despite a good dietary intake should be suspected of suffering from tuberculosis and treated accordingly. Failure to gain weight may also be due to HIV/AIDS.

Hypothermia

Malnourished children, particularly those who are marasmic, tend to have low body temperatures, especially at night. They must be kept warm, even if the air temperature seems uncomfortably warm to the staff. Encourage mothers to hold their children close to their bodies, against their skin, at night.

Very severe anaemia

If the haemoglobin concentration is less than 40 g/litre or the packed-cell volume is less than 12%, the child has very severe anaemia, which can cause heart failure. A child with very severe anaemia needs a blood transfusion. Give 10 ml of packed red cells or whole blood per kg of body weight *slowly* over 3 hours. Where testing for HIV and viral hepatitis B is not possible, transfusion should be given only when the haemoglobin concentration falls below 30 g/litre (or packed-cell volume below 10%), or when there are signs of life-threatening heart failure. Do *not* give iron during the initial phase of treatment, as it can have toxic effects and may reduce resistance to infection.

Lactose intolerance

In some regions (especially where there is no tradition of consumption of animal milks), profuse diarrhoea occurring immediately after a milk formula feed can be attributed to a low tolerance of the lactose in cow's milk. (Most diarrhoeas, however, are caused by infection.) Suspected lactose intolerance can be confirmed by withholding milk from a feed. If the diarrhoea is caused by milk, it will stop, and will start again when milk is reintroduced.

If lactose intolerance is confirmed, the milk in the feed can be replaced by sour milk, yoghurt, or a commercial lactose-free formula. If it is not confirmed, the milk-based diet can be continued.

Hypoglycaemia (low blood glucose)

Hypoglycaemia may be caused by a serious systemic infection or can occur when a malnourished child has not been fed for 4–6 hours. Hypoglycaemia is an important cause of death during the first 2 days. It is uncommon when feedings are given every 2–3 hours day and night. If hypoglycaemia is suspected (from low temperature, lethargy, and limpness) immediate treatment is needed. Treatment with a strong sugar solution (10% glucose or sucrose) or F-75 liquid formula given orally will be effective almost immediately. If necessary, sterile 10% glucose solution may be given intravenously (5 ml/kg body weight). This should be followed by frequent oral or nasogastric feedings of F-75 formula for a few days to prevent relapse.

Organizing a therapeutic feeding centre

Facilities

Therapeutic feeding centres can be set up in simple weatherproof shelters constructed from local materials. Each centre should be large enough to accommodate 50 children and their attendants (mothers or carers). It is better to build more than one shelter, if needed, than to have a single shelter that is too large. Each centre must have:

- enough water (30 litres per person per day)
- a kitchen with traditional stoves and fuel, and a storage room that is secure against theft
- latrines and washing facilities for the staff, patients, and attendants.

Equipment

Each therapeutic feeding centre will require the same basic equipment. As a rough guide, a centre that cares for 50 children will need the following:

- 50 beds (or mattresses or mats)
- 100 blankets
- 10 lanterns (with fuel) for staff and mothers (for night-time feeding)
- 5 cooking pots (with covers), local-style stoves, and enough fuel to prepare food six times a day
- 5 buckets, 5 stirrers, 5 measuring cups, food-weighing scales (up to 5 kg capacity)
- 100 feeding cups and spoons
- 25 nasogastric tubes with adhesive tape and 25 plastic 50-ml syringes
- 2 accurate weighing scales (hanging or beam-balance), and an adequate supply of growth charts, forms, pencils, pens, paper, measuring sticks, and length boards
- minimum standardized medical equipment and essential drugs for paediatric use.

Personnel

The centre will require enough personnel to maintain a round-the-clock feeding schedule. For the recommended number of about 50 resident children, the following are required:

- 1 experienced professional nurse/nutritionist, full-time
- 2 trained health workers
- 1 nursing aid for every 10 children
- 1 cleaner
- 2 cooks
- 1 storekeeper.

One doctor can visit up to 10 centres if travelling distances are small. A doctor's visit is necessary for overall supervision and to examine problem cases.

Personnel for the centre should be recruited from the affected population, and each helper should be trained to perform specific, well defined tasks.

Hygiene and food safety

Children suffering from PEM are very vulnerable to infections. To prevent infections:

- plenty of clean and safe water (at least 30 litres per person per day) must be available in the therapeutic feeding centre (and other health facilities);
- foods must be protected from flies, insects, and dust, and should not be reconstituted in advance;
- the mothers or other carers should clean the children's feeding plates and utensils after every meal;
- everyone who feeds the children must wash their hands with soap first;
- latrine facilities must be available for patients and personnel.

Further guidelines are given in Annex 5.

Record-keeping

Each child's progress should be carefully monitored and full records should be kept, including weight charts.

Treatment of severe wasting and famine oedema (adult kwashiorkor) in adolescents and adults

The principles of management of adolescents and adults with severe malnutrition and the physiological changes are the same as those in children. In general, the guidelines for management of children should be followed. There are, however, differences in the classification of malnutrition, the amount of food required, and the drug dosages.

Except in famine conditions, adolescents and adults rarely associate wasting or oedema with their diet. As a consequence, they do not believe that altering their diet will help them. Even in famine conditions, they are often very reluctant to eat anything except traditional foods, which they view as perfectly satisfactory. Moreover, the foods they are allowed are often restricted by cultural and religious beliefs. They are often reluctant to take formula feeds unless they can be persuaded that such feeds are a form of medicine. This problem is one of the most difficult aspects of treating adolescents and adults.

Adults with a BMI below 16.0 or with oedematous malnutrition should be admitted to a therapeutic feeding centre. If symmetrical oedema is present, its cause must be determined. In addition to malnutrition, causes in adults include pre-eclampsia (in pregnant women), severe proteinuria (nephrotic syndrome), nephritis, acute filariasis (the limb is hot and painful), heart failure, and wet

Table 28 Dietary requirements for initial treatment of severely malnourished adolescents and adults

Age (years)	Total energy requirement[a] (kcal$_{th}$/kg body weight per day)	Volume of diet (ml/kg body weight per hour)	
		F-75	F-100
7–10	75	4.2	3.0
11–14	60	3.5	2.5
15–18	50	2.8	2.0
19–75	40	2.2	1.7
>75	35	2.0	1.5

[a] Individual needs may vary by up to 30% from these figures.

beriberi. Non-nutritional causes of oedema can be readily identified by the history, physical examination, and urinalysis.

A thorough examination should be conducted to exclude conditions that give rise to secondary malnutrition. A careful dietary history should be taken. Blood sugar should be tested to exclude diabetes mellitus.

Initial treatment phase

If possible, adolescents and adults should be given the same formula feeds (with added minerals and vitamins) as children. The initial goal of treatment is to prevent further loss of tissue. The amount of feed given per kg of body weight is much less that for children and decreases with increasing age, reflecting the lower energy requirements of adults. Recommended amounts for different ages are given in Table 28. These amounts will meet all nutrient requirements of adolescents and adults. As most severely malnourished adults are anorexic, the formula is usually given by nasogastric tube during the first few days.

Adults and adolescents are also susceptible to hypothermia and hypoglycaemia. The latter condition is managed as described for children. They should also be given systemic antimicrobials and, except for pregnant women, a single dose of 200 000 IU of vitamin A orally.

Rehabilitation phase

An improving appetite indicates the beginning of rehabilitation. During rehabilitation it is usual for adolescents and adults to become very hungry, often refusing the formula feed and demanding enormous amounts of solid food. When this happens, a diet should be given that is based on traditional foods, but with added oil, mineral mix, and vitamin mix. Provide a wide variety of foods and allow the patients to eat as much as they want. If possible, continue to give the formula feed with the vitamin and mineral mixes between meals and at night. Present the formula feed as a medicine if necessary.

Criteria for discharge

Adolescents and adults can be discharged when they are eating well and gaining weight, they have a reliable source of nutritious food outside the feeding centre, and any other health problems have been diagnosed and treatment begun. Adults should continue to receive a supplemented diet as outpatients until their BMI reaches 18.5.

Failure to respond to treatment

Failure of adults and adolescents to respond to treatment is usually due to an unrecognized underlying illness, a nutrient deficiency, or refusal to follow the treatment regimen.

Fuller details on treatment of severely malnourished adults and adolescents may be found in the following publication:

- *Management of severe malnutrition: a manual for physicians and other senior health workers*. Geneva, World Health Organization, 1999.

CHAPTER 6

Prevention, treatment, and control of communicable diseases

Infectious diseases and malnutrition are closely linked: malnourished populations are more susceptible to most infections, and the severity of illness and the mortality rates are worse. Moreover, infections can result in a borderline nutritional status becoming frank malnutrition, particularly in young children.

Measures to prevent infection are therefore of prime importance in both the prevention and management of nutritional emergencies. Preventive measures can be considered in the following major categories:

- general health programme coordination
- immunization programmes
- prevention of micronutrient deficiencies
- prevention and treatment of other specific important diseases
- environmental health measures.

General health measures include the coordination and integration of local and national health services in emergency areas; development and use of standardized procedures for prevention and treatment; and organization of disease surveillance and reporting.

Immunization programmes are particularly important. Most countries have established programmes of immunization against tuberculosis, diphtheria, pertussis (whooping cough), tetanus, poliomyelitis, and measles. Immunization against measles is crucial in emergencies. Other important communicable diseases are diarrhoeal and respiratory infections, malaria, and various febrile and parasitic diseases.

Environmental health measures include the provision of adequate shelter and living space, adequate and potable water supplies, washing facilities, safe food-handling, adequate latrines, and facilities for disposal of solid waste. Effective environmental health measures are among the best forms of insurance against most of the communicable diseases.

Introduction

Although the provision of food is the first relief priority in nutritional emergencies, it is also crucial to organize programmes for the prevention and treatment of major important diseases, particularly since food itself can be a vehicle for disease transmission. Wherever the population density is high, and especially in refugee and displaced-person camps, communicable diseases are responsible for most mortality and morbidity. The most important diseases are usually measles, diarrhoeal diseases, and respiratory infections, but malaria, typhoid, and typhus are also highly significant in some regions. Infants, children, elderly and sick people, and pregnant women are generally the most severely affected.

Disease prevention, through prompt attention to immunization and to the various aspects of environmental health (habitat, safe water, sanitation facilities, etc.), should be a priority. Caring for large numbers of sick people makes it essential to concentrate on the most important diseases and to standardize diagnosis and treatment. Where numbers of trained health workers are limited, local people should be trained as paramedical and community health workers.

General disease-prevention measures

Coordination of health programme activities

Under emergency conditions there is a natural tendency to set up special health service systems, either locally in affected areas or on a regional or national scale. To some extent, this may be for the convenience of external support agencies, but it invariably leads to difficulties later on. The health services for the affected population groups tend to become vertical operations which may be relatively expensive, with additional logistic requirements, and which may be difficult to phase out once the emergency is over. Where possible, it is preferable to provide additional support to existing services from the outset, rather than setting up parallel but separate services.

External agencies should accept that this may lead to some delay in initial action, since local health personnel may require special ad hoc training in emergency procedures. In the long run, however, working with local and national health services will help to build their capacities and self-reliance. Emergency preparedness training, including nutritional aspects, should be introduced systematically in disaster-prone areas and countries. A number of special centres have already been established for this purpose and many countries have emergency preparedness focal points. These activities, in turn, should be an integral part of national health development plans and of capacity-building in the health sector, to reduce the need to depend on external interventions. The current emphasis is on building the management capacities of local and national health services through systematic training programmes for personnel at all levels of the health system.

Overall medical responsibilities lie with local health authorities, and external relief workers should adapt to local standards and procedures. Familiarity with local culture, disease patterns, and health service organization is important in this regard.

Most countries are committed to the ideals of primary health care and strengthening of district health services. A particularly important feature of primary health care is the participation of communities in developing their own health-care systems, which may involve the designation of village health committees, training of village health workers and traditional birth attendants, and so on. District health teams, established within the framework of district development, with decentralization of authority to the district level, will be better equipped to deal with an emergency than more fragmented and centralized systems.

It is therefore important for external relief agencies, including nongovernmental organizations, to familiarize themselves with the state of development of local health services and to aim to work within the established system rather than developing parallel services.

Standardized procedures and materials

Standardization of the procedures used for disease prevention and treatment is particularly important in an emergency, as is clear definition of the role of each relief agency involved. Standard procedures should be put in writing and should reflect government policy; all health personnel should be familiar with them. Guidelines established in earlier emergencies may be useful but will probably need adapting to the new circumstances.

The range of drugs used in camps or in health facilities for the affected population should be limited to the minimum needed for the management of common diseases.[1] Similarly, medical equipment should be simple, tough, and easily replaceable. Many prepacked kits of materials and equipment are available, which simplifies ordering and supply.

Health information system

The main objectives of the health information system are to provide early warning of epidemics and, more broadly, to evaluate the current health situation and health programme coverage and impact. Apart from nutritional disorders, the following areas should be monitored:

- common acute infectious diseases, especially diarrhoeal and respiratory diseases, measles, and malaria
- diseases with epidemic potential — meningitis, cholera, dysentery (shigellosis), hepatitis
- immunization programmes
- water supply and sanitation programmes
- conditions of housing/shelter
- energy and fuel resources
- food resources.

[1] The national list of essential drugs should be consulted.

Disease surveillance

A disease surveillance system should be organized in order to identify possible outbreaks of common diseases and to give the earliest possible warning of incidence of a new disease ("sentinel" cases). Disease surveillance is usually based on reports of cases seen at health facilities and by health workers. Systematic, community-based surveys of most diseases are difficult and rarely attempted under emergency conditions. When an outbreak occurs, its source should be investigated and measures taken to prevent both the spread of the disease concerned and any further outbreaks.

Surveillance reports

Dispensaries, clinics, maternal and child health centres, and other health posts should identify and record major causes of illness. For some diseases (e.g. measles) this is straightforward, but for others (e.g. diarrhoea, with or without blood in the stools) it is more difficult — though no less desirable — to identify the cause. The reporting system should include only those diseases or symptoms of major public health significance that are easy to treat or prevent (this may include nutritional diseases, such as PEM, xerophthalmia, scurvy, beriberi, and pellagra). A sample reporting form, which may be adapted to local needs, is shown in Fig. 13.

The sex and approximate age of patients, or a breakdown by sex and age-groups (<5 years, 5 years and over), should be recorded on surveillance reports. Reports should be completed carefully, recording a zero (not a dash) if no specific illness is detected; if blanks are left, others will be unsure whether no cases were observed or no information was available. Information should be analysed on site and trends plotted on a wall-chart. Reporting to the district health office should be done *at least* monthly, and any outbreak of disease should be reported immediately by the quickest means.

Surveillance systems should be set up as an integral part of an existing government health information system, and reports should be sent to local/district health authorities. These authorities should be encouraged (and assisted when necessary) to take both diagnostic and remedial action in the event of increases in disease prevalence or incidence. Reports may also be copied to a central authority with overall responsibility for the emergency, but the full involvement of local authorities is highly desirable. Since reports may give rise to a degree of controversy on occasion, they should be very carefully compiled and issued only with the agreement of all concerned authorities. It is particularly important that demographic information should be accurate, so that the magnitude of various problems, trends in prevalence, and so on can be assessed.

Mortality data

Mortality data are crucial: change in the death rate is one of the key indicators of the effect of a relief programme. This information may be difficult to collect; families may be reluctant to report deaths, fearing that their rations will be reduced. It may be easiest to monitor death rates by counting graves at the designated burial site.

Fig. 13 Disease surveillance reporting form for district, village, health centre, or camp

	Month, trimester, or year 1	2	3	4
A. Nutritional status				
1. *Infants:* low-birth-weight incidence, i.e. $\frac{\text{(no. of birthweights} < 2500\,\text{g)}}{\text{(total no. of live births)}} \times 100\%$	....	....	....	....
2. *Infants and children:* underweight (low weight-for-age) or wasted (low weight-for-height), i.e. $\frac{\text{(no. below median} - 2\text{SD)}}{\text{(no. weighed, } N\text{)}} \times 100\%$				
Infants, 0–11 months: Enter *N*:	....	....	....	....
Enter % underweight:	....	....	....	....
Children, 12–59 months: Enter *N*:	....	....	....	....
Enter % underweight:	....	....	....	....
B. Morbidity/mortality[1] Enter: no. of cases seen (no. of deaths)				
Diarrhoea	..... (.....)	..... (.....)	..... (.....)	..... (.....)
Cholera	..... (.....)	..... (.....)	..... (.....)	..... (.....)
Jaundice	..... (.....)	..... (.....)	..... (.....)	..... (.....)
Malaria	..... (.....)	..... (.....)	..... (.....)	..... (.....)
Measles	..... (.....)	..... (.....)	..... (.....)	..... (.....)
Neonatal tetanus	..... (.....)	..... (.....)	..... (.....)	..... (.....)
Diphtheria	..... (.....)	..... (.....)	..... (.....)	..... (.....)
Pertussis (whooping cough)	..... (.....)	..... (.....)	..... (.....)	..... (.....)
Poliomyelitis	..... (.....)	..... (.....)	..... (.....)	..... (.....)
Acute respiratory infection	..... (.....)	..... (.....)	..... (.....)	..... (.....)
Tuberculosis	..... (.....)	..... (.....)	..... (.....)	..... (.....)
Amoebiasis	..... (.....)	..... (.....)	..... (.....)	..... (.....)
Hookworm disease	..... (.....)	..... (.....)	..... (.....)	..... (.....)
Anaemia	..... (.....)	..... (.....)	..... (.....)	..... (.....)
Xerophthalmia	..... (.....)	..... (.....)	..... (.....)	..... (.....)
Goitre	..... (.....)	..... (.....)	..... (.....)	..... (.....)
Total no. of individuals seen (all conditions)	..... (.....)	..... (.....)	..... (.....)	..... (.....)

[1] Ideally, these data should be complemented by information on treatments given and deaths, for each category.

Deaths should be reported in terms of rate, i.e. the number of deaths per 10 000 people per day, or per 1000 people per month, depending on the severity of the situation. Age-specific mortality data (e.g. deaths among children under 5 years) should also be reported, weekly, monthly, or quarterly, and sex-specific death rates should be calculated as soon as the workload allows. For any of these rates to be calculated it is essential to know the total size of the population and the breakdown by age (at least in terms of <5 years and ≥5 years).

The crude mortality rate (number of deaths from all causes per 10 000 people per day) should not exceed 1/10 000; a rate of 2/10 000 indicates a severe situation.

Rates several times higher than this are not uncommon in emergencies. Among children under 5 years, a mortality rate of 1/10 000 indicates a serious situation, and 2/10 000 a severe situation. However, trends over time are more important than single results. The cause of any rising trend should be carefully investigated. Studies have shown, for instance, that mortality rates rise significantly when available food supplies provide an energy intake of less than 2000 $kcal_{th}$ per person per day.

Priority-setting and phasing

In the first 2–3 months of an emergency, it is unlikely that all medical problems can receive equal attention. The most frequent causes of death are likely to be malaria, diarrhoeal and respiratory disease, measles, and malnutrition. Tackling these disorders (and programmatic development such as measures for diarrhoeal disease control, maternal and child health, immunization, and environmental health) should take priority, possibly to the exclusion of other problems. When progress has been made in these areas, activities can be diversified.

Immunization — preventable diseases

Children who are both malnourished and living in overcrowded conditions are particularly susceptible to vaccine-preventable diseases, and special efforts must be made to immunize all such children as completely and as quickly as possible. In emergencies, attention should focus first on measles. Rapid, effective delivery of measles vaccine and vitamin A, in particular, may save large numbers of children from death or severe disability. As soon as possible, the national programme for childhood immunization must be (re-)established. In protracted and complex emergencies with low vaccine coverage, "mopping-up" campaigns for poliomyelitis may be used to complement the routine programme. Newborn infants should also be vaccinated with BCG whenever possible.

Women of childbearing age should be targeted for tetanus toxoid vaccination to prevent neonatal tetanus.

Almost all countries have established routine immunization programmes that cover at least tuberculosis, diphtheria, pertussis (whooping cough), tetanus, poliomyelitis, and measles: some also have programmes of immunization against yellow fever, viral hepatitis B, and meningitis. National immunization programmes generally follow the recommendations of WHO. Relief health coordinators should contact the national immunization programme to find out what services they can offer. Immunization provided as a part of relief efforts should be compatible with national policies and programmes.

Vaccine storage

Vaccines must be kept cold. Freeze-dried measles vaccine and oral poliomyelitis vaccine (OPV) are normally kept frozen at national and regional levels and at a temperature of 0–8 °C at other levels.

Now that all vials of OPV procured by WHO and UNICEF carry vaccine vial monitor (VVM) labels, health workers can, if necessary, continue to use vaccines where there is no cold chain or if icepacks have thawed. The VVM changes colour if a vial has been exposed to too high a temperature for too long, thus alerting the vaccinator. Once the colour change has occurred, the vial must not be used.

Reconstituted measles vaccine should be protected from direct sunlight, kept on ice during the immunization session, and not kept for more than 8 hours after reconstitution. It must never be kept overnight, even in a refrigerator. The liquid used for reconstitution must be that provided by the manufacturer of the vaccine and should be at a temperature of 0–8°C at the time of reconstitution to avoid thermal shock killing the virus.

Measles, meningitis, and poliomyelitis

Measles and meningitis outbreaks are especially dangerous in nutritional emergencies; they can spread rapidly and cause high death rates. Their prevention should receive urgent and particular attention.

Measles

Nutritional emergencies are likely to be precipitated by conditions such as refugee camps, which bring people into close contact, opening the way to rapid transmission of the measles virus. Malnourished children are at particularly high risk of complications and death following an attack of measles. The disease can trigger acute PEM (kwashiorkor) and worsen vitamin A deficiency in children whose nutritional status is already borderline.

Immunization is a priority measure during a nutritional emergency and, since speed is crucial, is generally carried out by relief agencies rather than by local health authorities. However, it is essential that the agencies consult fully with the local authorities.

There are no contraindications to measles immunization during emergencies: even if there is already a measles epidemic, immunization should continue. All children aged between 6 months and 5 years should be immunized when they are first registered or screened; this will ensure the earliest and most complete coverage and will prevent new arrivals from becoming infected. When measles vaccines are given before the age of 9 months, the scheduled dose of vaccine should also be given as soon as possible after infants reach 9 months of age (but with no less than 4 weeks between the two doses).

The upper age limit for measles immunization depends on local circumstances. If the population comes from a situation with high measles transmission and low immunization coverage over the previous 3–5 years, it is probably reasonable to vaccinate only children between the ages of 6 months and 5 years. However, if local health authorities cannot guarantee that the population has been recently exposed, or if the population originates from isolated and widely dispersed communities, the target group should be expanded to include children up to the age of 15 years. Although the risk of a child's dying from measles complications diminishes with age, the disease can be transmitted from older to younger children (seeding). Thus, older children who are thought to be under-immunized should be regarded as a potential risk for causing a measles outbreak and should be included in the immunization target group.

If high immunization coverage has already been achieved in the community, and there is no evidence of circulation of the virus, it may be decided that further immunization is unnecessary. With this single exception, however, WHO recommends that measles immunization be given the highest possible priority.

Meningitis

Meningitis is an acute inflammation of the membrane (meninges) that surrounds the brain and spinal cord and may be either bacterial or viral in origin. The bacterial form is the more serious, caused principally by *Neisseria meningitidis*. Cycles of bacterial (meningococcal) meningitis occur in both East and West Africa (the sub-Saharan "meningitis belt") and sometimes in other areas; death rates are high unless the disease is treated immediately with antimicrobials.

Routine immunization against meningococcal meningitis is not generally recommended following disasters because it lacks efficacy in young children and offers protection of only short duration. However, in areas such as the African meningitis belt, post-emergency surveillance for meningitis using a standard case definition should be routine. A meningitis incidence exceeding 15 per 100 000 per week for a period of 2 consecutive weeks has been shown to be predictive of an outbreak in populations of over 100 000. In refugee camps where the population is unknown or is usually less than 100 000, a rough indicator of an outbreak is a doubling of the baseline number of meningitis cases from one week to the next over a period of 3 weeks.

When an outbreak occurs, emphasis must be placed on careful surveillance, early diagnosis (confirmed by a laboratory if possible), immediate treatment of suspected cases, and immunization (if the disease is due to a susceptible type of *Neisseria*).

Decisions on age groups to immunize depend on those affected, although immunizing all children and young adults from 1 to 25 years old will usually protect most of the population at risk. Priority should be given first to the areas or populations with the highest incidence rates. The programme will require good logistic support (staff, vaccines, cold chain for vaccine storage, transport, etc.).

The value of chemoprophylaxis — giving drugs to prevent meningitis — is a matter of some controversy.

Poliomyelitis

If the affected community has benefited from a national immunization day within the previous 9 months, it may be reasonable to avoid further immunization against poliomyelitis. Otherwise, oral poliomyelitis vaccine should be administered to all children from birth to 5 years of age. Those for whom there are records showing three properly administered doses have already been given should receive an additional booster dose; all other children should be given one dose immediately and subsequent doses according to the national schedule.

Other vaccines

If immunization or re-immunization with other vaccines, such as DPT (diphtheria/pertussis/tetanus), is feasible, suitable opportunities should be sought for their systematic administration.

Prevention and treatment of specific important diseases

As many as 80% of the people who go to a health post or other health facility will have minor illnesses. To avoid the unnecessary use of scarce resources (medicine, personnel time) on these cases, a screening system should be set up. This should be designed to detect the most serious and difficult cases and arrange for their referral to professional health personnel, leaving paramedical staff — appropriately trained — to handle lesser or more routine problems.

Presumptive treatment may be used for many diseases that are common but difficult to diagnose. For instance, in an area where malaria is common, any person with a fever that has no other obvious cause — such as an abscess or a respiratory infection — should be treated for malaria.

Standard treatment guidelines should be agreed between the national authorities and all health agencies. The following are some general guidelines:

- Single-dose treatment should be used whenever possible.
- Patients should not be provided with large supplies of tablets.
- Mixtures of tablets should be avoided — one drug is usually sufficient.
- Injections are very useful for certain problems, and generally appreciated by patients, but they are sometimes dangerous and almost always expensive, and should not be used indiscriminately.
- Drugs formulated as syrups or sugar-coated pills are no more active than simple tablets, but may be 5–10 times more expensive; their use should be avoided.

Diarrhoeal diseases

Diarrhoea may be caused by various types of pathogens, including bacteria (such as *Escherichia coli*, and *Shigella*, *Salmonella*, *Vibrio*, and *Campylobacter* species), parasites such as *Giardia* and *Cryptosporidium* species, and enteric viruses (e.g. rotavirus). Malnourished populations are particularly vulnerable to these pathogens. Moreover, chronic or repeated diarrhoea can itself cause undernutrition and eventually lead to impairment of the immune system and susceptibility to other infections. A vicious cycle of diarrhoea and malnutrition can become established (see Fig. 14) and cause death in many cases.

In a great proportion of cases, episodes of diarrhoeal disease are caused by contaminated food and/or drinking-water. Of the 1500 million diarrhoeal episodes that occur each year, worldwide, in children under the age of 5 years (causing 3 million deaths), it is estimated that 70% are due to consumption of contaminated food — particularly weaning food. Contamination of food may have any of a number of causes, including contact with nightsoil, polluted water, flies, pests, domestic animals, unclean cooking utensils, and unsanitary food handling. Raw foods themselves may harbour pathogens, for instance if they originate from infected food animals or from an environment in which the pathogens are naturally present.

The risk of diarrhoea is significantly increased by two principal errors in food handling and preparation:

Fig. 14 Interaction of diarrhaea and malnutrition

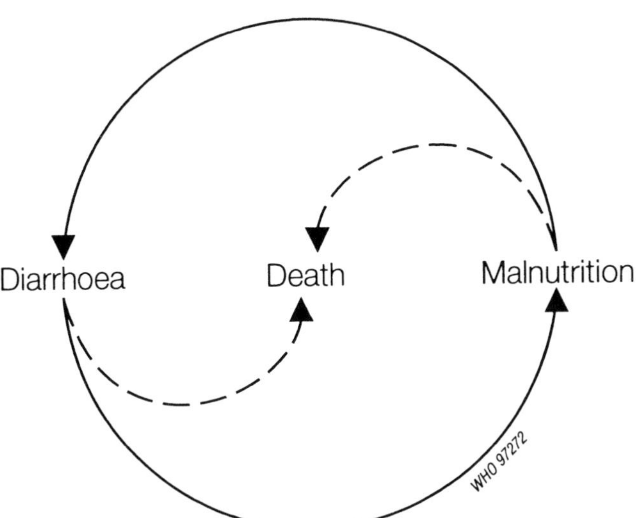

- preparation of food several hours in advance of its consumption, combined with storage at temperatures that favour growth of pathogenic bacteria and/or growth of bacteria to disease-causing levels;
- cooking or reheating food insufficiently to eliminate pathogens or reduce them to safe levels.

The approach to prevention of diarrhoea in developing countries is traditionally one of improving water supplies and sanitation. However, these measures alone are insufficient to solve the problem. The need for safe handling and preparation of food at household level should also be emphasized, and this calls for intensive education in food safety. In this regard, it is valuable to analyse the hazards associated with local food preparation traditions and to identify practices that should be modified.

The most important measures in the management of diarrhoeal diseases are:

- prevention or treatment of dehydration
- continued feeding (including breast-feeding) during the diarrhoeal episode
- monitoring of the condition of the patient.

The following publications deal in detail with the management of diarrhoeal diseases:

- *The treatment of diarrhoea: a manual for physicians and other senior health workers*. Geneva, World Health Organization, 1995 (unpublished WHO document WHO/CDR/95.3).[1]
- *The management of bloody diarrhoea in young children*. Geneva, World Health Organization, 1994 (unpublished WHO document WHO/CDD/94.49).[1]

[1] Available on request from Child and Adolescent Health and Development, World Health Organization, 1211 Geneva 27, Switzerland.

- *Guidelines for the control of epidemics due to* Shigella dysenteriae *type 1*. Geneva, World Health Organization, 1995 (unpublished WHO document WHO/CDR/95.4).[1]
- *Guidelines for cholera control*. Geneva, World Health Organization, 1993.
- *The clinical management of cholera*. Geneva, World Health Organization, 1991 (unpublished WHO document WHO/CDD/SER/91.45).[1]
- *Integrated management of childhood illness*. Geneva, World Health Organization (unpublished documents WHO/CHD/97.3A–M).[2]

Viral hepatitis

Five types of viral hepatitis are now recognized — A, B, C, D, and E. Acute hepatitis of any type can cause severe anorexia, nausea, vomiting, dehydration, and weight loss, and may last several weeks. Two forms — type A (formerly called infectious hepatitis) and type E (formerly called enterically transmitted non-A non-B hepatitis) — may be transmitted by contaminated water or food and can give rise to large-scale outbreaks or epidemics. Types B, C, and D are not transmitted by food or water but by contamination from blood or serous fluids.

Viral hepatitis A is usually endemic in developing countries with poor sanitation; most children are asymptomatically infected during the first few years of life and develop lifelong immunity. Epidemics are therefore rare in these countries and the principal threat is to individuals coming from industrialized countries. In the event of community disruption (war, natural disaster, etc.) in more developed countries, where many people are susceptible, epidemics of viral hepatitis A are common; infected food-handlers are frequently efficient vectors for transmission of the virus. The disease is rarely fatal and does not result in chronic hepatitis or a carrier state.

Control of viral hepatitis A depends on improving food sanitation and on purification or boiling of water. Immune globulin (gamma-globulin) is sometimes used to protect contacts of cases in households or institutions but is rarely effective in controlling community-wide outbreaks. An inactivated hepatitis A vaccine is now available and highly effective in protecting individuals; it has also been proved effective for the control of widespread outbreaks of the disease, but is too expensive for routine public health use.

Large outbreaks of waterborne viral hepatitis E occur in areas where sanitation is poor, and epidemics of acute hepatitis in developing countries are more likely to be due to hepatitis E than A. The virus has been responsible for large epidemics in refugee camps and among displaced and disrupted population groups. Symptoms are similar to those of viral hepatitis A, and no chronic disease or carrier state develops as a result of infection; however, as many as 20% of pregnant women who develop symptomatic disease in the third trimester will die from

[1] Available on request from Emerging Diseases, World Health Organization, 1211 Geneva 27, Switzerland.

[2] Available on request from Child and Adolescent Health and Development, World Health Organization, 1211 Geneva 27, Switzerland.

fulminant hepatitis. There is no vaccine and no evidence of immune globulin having any protective efficacy; the only known preventive measure is the provision of safe water. There is no specific treatment.

Malaria

Like other infections, malaria readily causes nutritional deterioration in both children and adults, especially when it is recurrent. Specifically, the haemolysis associated with acute malaria causes anaemia, which becomes chronic, particularly if — as is often the case — there is an associated deficiency of iron and/or folate. During a malaria epidemic the entire non-immune population is at risk of serious disease.

Protection of pregnant women against malaria is particularly important because of the risks of anaemia, abortion, stillbirth, and premature delivery, especially in a first pregnancy. The risks of spontaneous abortion and of maternal mortality as a result of malaria are up to 60% and 10%, respectively, in non-immune pregnant women. Infants born to infected mothers are likely to be of low birth weight and may be anaemic (or become so subsequently).

In view of the high maternal and infant morbidity and the mortality associated with malaria in pregnancy, intermittent treatment with an effective, preferably one-dose, antimalarial drug, delivered in the context of antenatal care, should be made available to primigravidae and secundigravidae as an appropriate and effective method of reducing the consequences of malaria in pregnancy in highly endemic areas. Such intermittent treatment should be given from the second trimester onwards, at intervals of *at least* 1 month.

For young children, WHO's recommendations are generally for early and effective treatment rather than regular prophylaxis. In any given setting, however, national guidelines for malaria prevention and treatment should be followed; a number of general principles are outlined in the following paragraphs.

Prevention

Prevention of malaria is by vector control and chemoprophylaxis. The objective of vector control is to reduce malaria morbidity and mortality by reducing levels of transmission. The measures employed will depend on local epidemiological, ecological, social, and economic characteristics, but may include:

- personal protection — bednets, curtains, eave strips,[1] window and door screens, etc., all impregnated with long-acting insecticides;
- indoor residual spraying, which will vary in efficacy according to house structure and the type of surface sprayed;
- larval control and environmental management in areas where mosquito breeding sites are well defined.

Effective vector control depends on a number of factors:

- planning to ensure that development activities do not exacerbate the malaria problem (by creating pools of standing water for example);

---

[1] Strips of cloth placed over openings between roof and walls to prevent entry of mosquitos.

- community participation in filling in abandoned wells, borrow pits, and other places where water may accumulate and provide breeding sites;
- large-scale environmental activities, such as draining of marshlands, and sound agricultural practices.

Chemoprophylaxis can no longer be considered a principal means of preventing malaria because of the spread of drug resistance, although it is still desirable for non-immune visitors to endemic areas. Drug choice depends on the sensitivity of parasites in a particular location and should therefore be based on national, rather than international, guidelines.

Treatment

Early diagnosis and prompt treatment of malaria will shorten the duration of the disease and prevent both complications and the majority of deaths. Where malaria is present, laboratory facilities for rapid diagnosis combined with standardized care protocols can greatly reduce the impact of the disease. This is particularly important for detecting both severe and, in areas of unstable or low transmission, uncomplicated disease, and for identifying treatment failures. These facilities are essential where both *Plasmodium vivax* and *P. falciparum* occur and recommended therapies for the two infections are different.

Treatment should be administered according to national drug policy, which is defined according to criteria of drug efficacy, safety, costs, and patient compliance. More detailed information on the most commonly used drugs and on the management of complicated and uncomplicated malaria and malaria in pregnancy may be found in the following publications:

- *Antimalarial drug policies: data requirements, treatment of uncomplicated malaria, and management of malaria in pregnancy.* Geneva, World Health Organization, 1994 (unpublished WHO document WHO/MAL/94.1070).[1]
- *Management of uncomplicated malaria and the use of antimalarial drugs for the protection of travellers.* Geneva, World Health Organization, 1997 (unpublished WHO document WHO/MAL/96.1075 Rev.1).[1]
- *Management of severe malaria: a practical handbook*, 2nd ed. Geneva, World Health Organization, 2000.

Acute respiratory infections

Acute respiratory infections (ARI) are the largest single immediate cause of mortality in childhood in developing countries. Malnutrition is an important risk factor for the development of ARI (and many other communicable diseases): malnourished children and adults with a cough are more likely to develop pneumonia, and the case-fatality rate in pneumonia is higher among malnourished individuals. In addition, the anorexia, breathing difficulties, and fever that may accompany ARI often result in weight loss during and immediately after each episode.

---

[1] Available on request from Malaria Control, World Health Organization, 1211 Geneva 27, Switzerland.

The most important cause of death from ARI is pneumonia, most cases of which can be detected by clinical assessment. Young children with coughs or breathing difficulties should be examined for fast breathing and chest indrawing. Fast breathing is a sensitive sign of pneumonia in children; the rate should be counted over 60 seconds and the following thresholds should be considered as indicative of pneumonia requiring antimicrobial therapy:

- for infants up to 2 months of age — 60 breaths per minute
- for infants aged from 2 up to 12 months — 50 breaths per minute
- for children from 12 months up to 5 years — 40 breaths per minute.

Severe infection causes stiffening of the lungs and chest indrawing: the lower chest wall moves in as the child breathes in. Any child with this sign should be referred urgently for skilled care where oxygen and second-line antimicrobials are available. Infants up to 2 months of age who show either fast breathing or chest indrawing should be retained.

Children aged 2 months to 5 years

The most important causes of pneumonia in children are *Streptococcus pneumoniae* and *Haemophilus influenzae*. Most cases can be treated on an outpatient basis with a 5-day course of oral co-trimoxazole (trimethoprim–sulfamethoxazole), amoxicillin, or ampicillin. Severe cases (e.g. young children with chest indrawing, or infants under 2 months of age with fast breathing or chest indrawing) are best treated with intramuscular benzylpenicillin, given 6-hourly, when admission to hospital is possible; otherwise amoxicillin is the most useful oral antibiotic. Gentamicin should be added to the penicillin for the treatment of young infants.

In the presence of clinically severe malnutrition (marasmus, kwashiorkor, or marasmic kwashiorkor), signs of pneumonia may be less obvious. Coughing and breathing difficulties in these circumstances should be treated on an inpatient basis whenever possible; chloramphenicol is the most appropriate treatment.

Infants under 2 months of age

Young infants can rapidly become very sick with pneumonia and may well die: in many developing countries, 20–30% of all deaths from ARI among children under 5 years old occur in the first 2 months of life. All young infants with any sign of pneumonia or other sepsis should be referred to a hospital for treatment with benzylpenicillin and gentamicin. If this is not possible, chloramphenicol can be used at a reduced dose (25 mg/kg body weight, 12-hourly) except in premature or low-birth-weight infants. It is also possible to use co-trimoxazole, ampicillin, or amoxicillin if this is all that is available, but co-trimoxazole should be avoided in premature or jaundiced neonates.

Supportive home care

Supportive home care, in addition to treatment with antimicrobials, is important, and should follow the guidelines of the national ARI programme, which generally recommends:

- continued feeding
- adequate fluid intake
- use of safe and appropriate cough/cold remedies
- prompt referral in the event of deterioration
- in young infants, avoidance of chilling.

Prevention

Childhood pneumonia can be largely prevented in emergencies if: nutritional status is maintained; immunization rates against measles and pertussis are kept high; overcrowding, poor ventilation, and smoky cooking fires are controlled; and early treatment of cough and breathing difficulties is sought and provided.

Treatment

Details of the management of acute respiratory infections may be found in the following publications:

- *The management of acute respiratory infections in children: practical guidelines for outpatient care*. Geneva, World Health Organization, 1995.
- *Outpatient management of young children with acute respiratory infections: a four-day clinical course*. Geneva, World Health Organization, 1995 (unpublished WHO document WHO/CDR/95.10).[1]
- *Acute respiratory infections in children: case management in small hospitals in developing countries. A manual for doctors and other senior health workers*. Geneva, World Health Organization, 1990 (unpublished WHO document WHO/ARI/90.5).[1]
- *Integrated management of childhood illness*. Geneva, World Health Organization (unpublished WHO documents WHO/CHD/97.3A–M).[1]

Measles

Immunization against measles also offers the best protection against complications of the disease. If complications do arise, active supportive treatment is essential to avoid death rates of 15–20% (or higher). All children with measles should therefore be given high-dose vitamin A supplements. Doses are given in Tables 15 and 16 in Chapter 2; oral vitamin A capsules are effective — there is no need to use injectable preparations of the vitamin. The following approach is recommended:

- First dose immediately on diagnosis, with a second dose the following day. The reason for the second dose is to ensure that body stores of vitamin A are built up again, even if a child has diarrhoea and is very ill.
- A child with clinical signs of vitamin A deficiency (such as Bitot's spots) should receive a third dose at least 2 weeks later.

---

[1] Obtainable on request from Child and Adolescent Health and Development, World Health Organization, 1211 Geneva 27, Switzerland.

- Mothers should be instructed about the importance of vitamin A and about its administration, since the second dose can be given at home (thus avoiding a second visit to the health facility and the risk of infecting other children).
- Mothers should also be advised about the importance of feeding their children locally available vitamin A-rich foods.

A standard approach to the management of measles should include treatment for respiratory complications, diarrhoea, potentially blinding eye lesions, and otitis media. Pneumonia can be treated effectively with an antimicrobial. Ampicillin, amoxicillin, or co-trimoxazole should be given; if none of these is available, procaine penicillin should be given for 5 days. The child should return for reassessment after 2 days — or sooner if the condition worsens. Diarrhoea may require oral rehydration therapy. Children who develop eye complications should be given antimicrobial eye ointments and a further dose of vitamin A after 14–21 days. (Eye ointments containing steroids should never be used to treat eye complications of measles.) Otitis media should also respond to antimicrobials.

The case-fatality rate from measles is very high in malnourished children and measles can precipitate severe malnutrition. It is therefore important to monitor nutritional status following measles and ensure that children eat and drink even if they have no appetite, are vomiting, or have diarrhoea. Mothers should be taught the importance of feeding sick children both during and after illness.

Meningitis

Bacterial meningitis can be treated with penicillin, ampicillin, or chloramphenicol; the drug should be selected according to the local treatment schedule. Treatment must be started as early as possible in the course of the disease; if this can be done, deaths from the most common types of bacterial meningitis can be reduced to less than 10%.

It is crucial to monitor and report weekly on any new cases of meningitis, and the establishment of a meningitis task force is highly desirable.

Tuberculosis

The global burden of tuberculosis is growing with increasing poverty, overcrowding, multiple-drug resistance, and the spread of HIV infection. In emergencies, all these factors are liable to be operating, together with poor nutritional status. The consequent weakening of the immune system, combined with malnutrition, directly affects the outcome of tuberculosis, leading to death within 5 years in 50% of cases and chronic infectious tuberculosis in 25%. Inadequately treated tuberculosis itself can cause moderate or severe malnutrition (cachexia, marasmus) in both adults and children.

WHO has developed and adopted a new strategy for effective tuberculosis control, known as DOTS — Directly Observed Treatment, Short course — and based on implementation of the following measures through primary health care:

- case-finding among tuberculosis suspects by sputum smear microscopy in general health services;

- standardized short-course chemotherapy in at least all smear-positive cases;
- directly observed treatment of the initial phase (first 60 doses) of chemotherapy;
- regular and uninterrupted supply of essential anti-tuberculosis drugs;
- monitoring system for programme supervision and evaluation.

In emergency situations, case management can usefully include food supplements, which will hasten recovery and provide needed support to affected families. In children, especially those who are malnourished, susceptibility both to infection and to progress of infection to disease is enhanced. Malnourished children of all ages are therefore considered to be at risk of developing severe active tuberculosis.

Prevention

The main methods of tuberculosis prevention are:

- early diagnosis and effective cure of infectious cases of tuberculosis;
- BCG vaccination, usually of newborns; vaccination is also strongly recommended for children up to age 5 years who have never been vaccinated and who are not suffering from other diseases (e.g. AIDS), but revaccination is not recommended;
- screening of contacts (especially those under 6 years of age) of infectious, smear-positive cases of pulmonary tuberculosis.

Treatment

Details of treatment of tuberculosis may be found in the following publications:

- WHO/UNHCR. *Tuberculosis control in refugee situations: an interagency field manual.* Geneva, World Health Organization, 1997 (unpublished WHO document WHO/TB/97.221).[1]
- *Treatment of tuberculosis: guidelines for national programmes*, 2nd ed. Geneva, World Health Organization, 1997 (unpublished WHO document WHO/TB/97.220).[1]
- Grafton J. *Guidelines for the management of drug-resistant tuberculosis.* Geneva, World Health Organization, 1997 (unpublished WHO document WHO/TB/96.210 (Rev.1)).[1]

Louse-borne typhus

Epidemic (louse-borne) typhus is a severe febrile disease caused by *Rickettsia prowazekii*, which is transmitted to humans by the body louse. It often occurs in overcrowded conditions where hygiene and sanitation are poor, and is therefore a significant risk in refugee camps and similar situations. Control of lice is the most effective means of preventing the disease, and the following measures are recommended:

[1] Obtainable on request from Global Tuberculosis Programme, World Health Organization, 1211 Geneva 27, Switzerland.

- application of a residual insecticide; dusting 0.5% permethrin powder on clothing is usually effective, but a safe alternative should be found if lice are resistant;
- immunization of susceptible individuals entering typhus areas, which may be feasible in some countries;
- provision of bathing and clothes-washing facilities.

Typhoid fever

Typhoid fever is an acute illness caused by *Salmonella typhi*, which is usually ingested with food or water that has been contaminated by the faeces of an infected person or a carrier. The best preventive measure is cleanliness — safe food and water and adequate facilities for personal hygiene. Infected individuals should not handle food and should be isolated from others while under treatment.

Scabies

Scabies is an eruption of the skin, with intense itching, caused by the mite *Sarcoptes scabiei*. Mites can spread from person to person and lesions may become infected. Affected people should be treated immediately, to prevent the spread of scabies. Clothing should be boiled, if possible, and all members of a family affected by the infestation should be treated at the same time.

Treatment consists of the application of 25% benzyl benzoate to the entire body, from the neck down. It should be applied on two consecutive nights and washed off 24 hours after the second application. When benzyl benzoate is contraindicated (in children, or men with eczema of the scrotum) treatment should be with permethrin, 5% cream or 1% lotion. Sulfur ointment in paraffin (concentration 10% for adults, 2% for children) can be used for pregnant women and children.

Worm infections

Worms in the intestine consume a significant portion of the food intake and contribute to malnutrition. Roundworm and hookworm infections are particularly common.

Roundworm

Roundworms (*Ascaris lumbricoides*) often cause no symptoms and their presence may not be suspected until they are seen in the stools or expelled through the mouth or nose. If microscopy facilities are available, eggs may be observed in stool samples. A heavy infestation may impair nutrition by provoking recurrent respiratory infections and, occasionally, causing intestinal obstruction.

Sanitary latrines, personal cleanliness, and hygienic food handling are important for preventing infection. However, intestinal parasitic infections may also arise from direct environmental contact, for instance with soil, clothes, or foods (such as vegetables) that are contaminated with the infective stages of the parasites. Infections are commonly caused by consumption of contaminated raw vegetables in tropical countries (see also Chapter 4). If the infection is widespread, mass treatment of all children should be instituted, giving a single dose of an anthelminthic (albendazole, levamisole, mebendazole, or pyrantel). A single dose of one of these drugs can also be used for individual treatment of *Ascaris* infection.[1]

Hookworm

Hookworm (*Ancylostoma* sp. and *Necator americanus*) infection may give rise to few overt symptoms or may cause abdominal pain, iron deficiency anaemia, and other symptoms, depending on the number of worms in the body. Control of the problem depends largely on the provision of sanitary facilities.

Where infections, and attendant anaemia, are common, single doses of albendazole, levamisole, mebendazole, or pyrantel (which are also active against roundworms) can be used for treatment, together with iron therapy (as described elsewhere in this manual).[1]

Human immunodeficiency virus (HIV) and acquired immunodeficiency syndrome (AIDS)

The characteristics and associated findings of symptomatic HIV infection are summarized in the following documents:

- *Guidelines for the clinical management of HIV infection in adults.* Geneva, World Health Organization, 1991 (unpublished WHO document WHO/GPA/IDS/HCS/91.6).[2]
- *Guidelines for the clinical management of HIV infection in children.* Geneva, World Health Organization, 1993 (unpublished WHO document WHO/GPA/IDS/HCS/93.3).[2]
- *Guidelines for HIV interventions in emergency settings.* Geneva, Joint United Nations Programme on HIV/AIDS, 1996 (unpublished document UNAIDS/96.1).[2]

These documents also give summary guidelines for the laboratory diagnosis of HIV infection. Further details are available in:

- WHO/Joint United Nations Programme on HIV/AIDS. Revised recommendations for the selection and use of HIV antibody tests. *Weekly epidemiological record*, 1997, 72(12):81–87.

Loss of weight or, in children, failure to gain weight, in HIV infections is the result of several mechanisms:

- inadequate nutritional intake as a result of anorexia or dysphagia, due to various factors:
  - — HIV-related oropharyngeal lesions, oesophagitis, or gastritis

---

[1] General guidelines on the use of drugs for parasitic diseases may be found in: *WHO model prescribing information: drugs used in parasitic diseases*, Geneva, World Health Organization, 1990, and *WHO informal consultation on the use of chemotherapy for the control of morbidity due to soil-transmitted nematodes in humans*, Geneva, World Health Organization, 1996 (unpublished WHO document WHO/CTD/SIP/96.2, available on request from Communicable Diseases Control, Prevention and Eradication, World Health Organization, 1211 Geneva 27, Switzerland).

[2] Available on request from Joint United Nations Programme on HIV/AIDS, 1211 Geneva 27, Switzerland.

— other intercurrent infections

— other deficiencies (e.g. iron, zinc), which induce anorexia

— physical weakness, anxiety, depression, HIV-related disorders of the central nervous system

— medication for HIV or related infections;

- malabsorption of macronutrients and micronutrients as a result of mucosal damage, diarrhoea, and infection of the gastrointestinal tract;
- intrinsic metabolic factors, including increased energy expenditure and protein catabolism as a result of fever caused by HIV or other infections.

Studies in HIV-infected adults have shown that weight loss in malnutrition is primarily a loss of both lean body mass and fat. The relationship that exists between weight loss, depletion of lean mass, and survival suggests that the timing of death is related to the extent of the loss of lean mass. Moreover, studies in asymptomatic patients have shown early changes in body composition and metabolism and indicated that nutritional state (including growth failure in children) influences survival independently of changes in CD4 lymphocyte counts. In the early, asymptomatic stages of disease, these metabolic changes are reversible; later, they become irreversible.

Micronutrient status (including vitamins A, B_1, B_2, B_6, and B_{12}, folate, iron, zinc, and selenium) is commonly impaired in HIV infection. Iron deficiency anaemia and lymphocytopenia are characteristic of the symptomatic disease. These deficiencies — particularly of vitamin A and zinc — may contribute to susceptibility to HIV infection, progress from asymptomatic to symptomatic disease, and further progress to severe disease and death.

The general nutritional management of AIDS patients does not differ fundamentally from that of other malnourished individuals. The major aim is to minimize loss of lean body mass and prevent micronutrient deficiencies in adults, and to maintain normal growth and micronutrient status in children. Oral feeding is always the first choice, with enteral or parenteral feeding only when necessary. Once nutritional deterioration has set in, it is difficult to check its progress; thus, ensuring adequate dietary intakes in the early stages of disease can prolong life. Some studies indicate that boosting BMI substantially above average levels (to values of 22–25) is beneficial.

Because of problems of malabsorption, it has been suggested that micronutrient intake should be increased, where feasible, by a factor of between 2 and 6. If HIV medication, which has anti-folate action, is used, folate supplements should be given. Where there are oropharyngeal and gastrointestinal lesions, meals should be soft or semi-liquid and non-irritant. Special efforts are needed to maintain energy and protein intakes; small, frequent meals should be encouraged. Fats and oils are poorly tolerated and are not recommended as a means of boosting energy-density of meals, and meals should also be low in lactose, fibre, and residue. In more advanced disease with chronic complications, especially chronic diarrhoea with small or large bowel disease, specific dietary modifications are recommended, based on the principles of management of other chronic diseases and on experience of their use in AIDS patients. Details may be found in:

- Guidelines for nutrition support in AIDS. *Cajanus*, 1996, 29(2):62–83.

Food supplements should be provided for wasted AIDS patients just as for other individuals with severe malnutrition; there is no justification for discrimination. In a community substantially affected by AIDS, it is preferable to provide food supplements to the entire community rather than to particular individuals or families.

Integrated management of childhood illness

Pneumonia, diarrhoea, malaria, measles, and malnutrition are responsible for more than 70% of the deaths of children under 5 years of age in developing countries and in emergency situations, and both this chapter and Chapter 5 have discussed various aspects of management of these diseases. Health workers have experience in treating the common illnesses of childhood, but are often trained in disease-specific approaches. In emergencies, they are likely to be confronted with large numbers of very sick children with multiple problems. They may then have difficulty in deciding which of the presenting signs and symptoms are the most important, which disorder to treat first if a child has more than one, and how to apply the various guidelines. Health workers must also bear in mind the relationships that exist between different disorders, for example recurrent diarrhoea and malnutrition.

Effective management in these circumstances calls for good diagnostic, therapeutic, and counselling skills. In recent years, a systematic process that deals with case management through a series of algorithms and guidelines has been developed by WHO and UNICEF. It is referred to as "integrated management of childhood illness" (IMCI), and describes the essential processes in sequence:

1. Assess and classify the sick child.
2. Identify and provide appropriate treatment.
3. Counsel the mother.

The processes deal separately with children in two age groups — from 1 week up to 2 months and from 2 months up to 5 years. They include procedures for assessment of the nutritional status of all children and of dietary practices (breast-feeding, complementary feeding) for children who are under 2 years old, who are underweight for age, or who have feeding problems. All the guidelines are based on existing WHO recommendations for the management of these disorders. Training modules are available to assist in the training of trainers and of staff at the health-centre level,[1] and complementary guidelines for the management of children needing referral are being developed.

The charts are generic in nature and need to be adapted to the local epidemiological and health-service situation before they can be used in any particular country. Many countries are now embarking on such a process with a view to using the guidelines as the basis for first-level child care.

---

[1] Unpublished WHO document series WHO/CHD/97.3 A–M, available on request from Child and Adolescent Health and Development, World Health Organization, 1211 Geneva 27, Switzerland.

By covering the most important diseases of childhood, the guidelines are particularly relevant to the acute emergency situation, but they also address long-term aspects of disease prevention and health promotion, making them relevant to situations with chronic problems. Health workers fully trained in IMCI will provide more effective clinical care for the sick child than those with more restricted training.

As IMCI is more widely adopted, locally adapted guidelines will be available that can be used as the standard for care in emergency situations. This will facilitate the selection of essential drugs for emergency supplies and the standardization of treatment given by all concerned in an emergency. The longer-term aspects of IMCI will provide a basis for the development of first-line health services for refugees. The introduction of this initiative thus has considerable potential as an element of emergency preparedness.

Environmental health

Good environmental health — in the areas of general habitat, water supplies, and sanitation facilities — is a basic requirement in all communities, including camps for displaced people. It is crucial for preventing many problems, yet is frequently ignored.

Shelter

Housing and general environmental conditions can have an important bearing on the outcome of emergency situations, especially as determinants of many diseases, notably those discussed in this chapter. In large-scale or countrywide emergencies it is impossible to make much change in these conditions in the short term but their importance should still be borne in mind with a view to appropriate improvements during the rehabilitation phase.

The creation of camps for refugees and other displaced populations should be avoided as far as possible, but where they exist already or have to be established (even if only temporarily), health aspects of the habitat they provide are a paramount consideration. Selection of appropriate sites should take account of the following factors:

- availability and accessibility of adequate water sources or existing drinking-water supply systems;
- proximity of land suitable for agriculture (avoiding steep slopes and land prone to erosion);
- soil characteristics (digging of latrines) and topography (drainage of waste-water);
- physical accessibility of the area (roads, bridges, etc.);
- accessibility of local markets;
- facilities for solid waste disposal.

With regard to the housing environment, a number of features that have important direct or indirect effects on the physical and mental health of occupants have been identified:

- structure, including protection offered against extremes of temperature, noise, dust, rain, insects, and rodents;
- qualitative and quantitative adequacy of water supplies;
- facilities for disposal and subsequent management of excreta and liquid and solid wastes;
- safety of the site, in terms of drainage, protection from contamination, etc;
- avoidance of overcrowding as a means of limiting the potential for accidents and the spread of disease;
- indoor pollution from the fuel used for cooking and heating;
- facilities for food storage (to avoid spoilage, infestation with insects, etc.);
- existence of disease vectors and hosts;
- use of the home as a workplace, which may involve storage and use of hazardous materials or equipment.

Further details on the implications of the habitat for health may be found in *Our planet, our health.*[1]

In the relief phase, and subsequently, it should be feasible to mobilize food aid (food-for-work) in support of improvement to the habitat and general environment in a camp along similar lines to those indicated in the broader context of Chapter 7 of this manual. The main constraint may be finding the materials and financial support for such activities but, with careful planning from the outset, they should be available by the time the rehabilitation phase begins.

Water supply

It is equally important to ensure the safety of water and provide adequate quantities. The amount of water needed by each person varies with the setting, but the following are the approximate needs:

Location / circumstances	*Volume per person per day*
Clinics, field hospitals	40–60 litres
Feeding centres	30 litres
Personal needs	15–20 litres

Water should be collected from the cleanest available source. In the case of a well, installation of a simple pulley device and provision of buckets will make raising the water easier. Water sources should be protected by the following measures:

- A fence or wall should be erected to keep animals away.
- Drainage ditches should be dug uphill from an open well to prevent storm water flowing into it.
- People should not be allowed to wash in the water source; children should not be allowed to play in or around a source.

---

[1] *Our planet, our health.* Geneva, World Health Organization, 1992 (Chapter 7).

- Latrines should not be located (or defecation allowed) uphill from or within 30 metres of a water source.

In addition, families should be instructed to:

- collect and store water in clean containers;
- empty and clean out containers regularly;
- keep each storage container covered and not allow children or animals to drink directly from a container;
- prevent people (particularly children) from putting their hands into the containers;
- take water from a container using a dipper kept specially for the purpose.

Water can be made safe by chemical treatment, commonly chlorine and chlorine-releasing compounds. These are available in several forms:

- bleaching powder (25% by weight of available chlorine when fresh); this deteriorates quickly when stored in warm and damp places;
- calcium hypochlorite (typically 70% by weight of available chlorine); this is more stable than bleaching powder;
- sodium hypochlorite (normally sold as a solution of strength approximately 5%).

The chlorine dose should be carefully determined, and it may be necessary to seek the advice of sanitation experts. Moreover, the indiscriminate distribution of chlorine tablets usually does little good and may actually be harmful (the tablets are dangerous if swallowed).

Where chemicals are not available, water may be boiled for 1 minute to kill harmful organisms. If the local water source is known to be contaminated, it may be possible to arrange for large quantities of clean drinking-water to be brought from elsewhere in drums or tank-trucks.

When it seems likely that emergency conditions will persist for some time, more permanent facilities should be sought urgently, including artesian wells, boreholes, and pumping and filtration equipment. In any case it is essential to disinfect water, either at the source in the case of centralized production or in the household by chlorination or boiling.

Further details on water supplies in emergency situations may be found in:

- *Water manual for refugee situations*. Geneva, Office of the United Nations High Commissioner for Refugees, 1992.

Environmental sanitation

Latrines must be provided wherever large groups of people are living together. An education programme should be conducted to explain why and how the latrines should be used. Ideally, one latrine should be constructed for each family.

Two common types of latrine are the ventilated improved pit (VIP) latrine (with vent pipe) and the pour-flush latrine (which is flushed by pouring into it about 3 litres of water after each defecation). Other types of latrine are described below.

Whenever latrines are provided, they should be:

- easy to reach at night;
- cleaned at least daily (people will not use dirty latrines); staff may have to be employed for this;
- sited well away from sources of drinking-water (at a distance of at least 30 metres) and 1.5–3 m above the water table).

Families should be instructed to keep latrines clean by regularly washing down dirty surfaces. If there are no latrines, defecation fields should be organized as an emergency measure while the latrines are being built. These fields should be established at least 30 m away from any source of drinking-water. Families should be instructed to:

- defecate away from houses or shelters, paths, and areas where children play, and at least 30 m away from a water source;
- avoid going barefoot to defecate;
- prevent children from going to the defecation area alone.

The deep-trench latrine

The deep-trench latrine is designed for camps that are set up to last several months. It consists of a trench 2–4 m deep and 75–90 cm wide; its length depends on the number of users, but should provide 1 m for each place, and 1 place for every 4–5 people. A deep trench should be shored up to prevent collapse, and should be covered with a fly-proof floor made of strong pieces of wood or bamboo that overlap the edges of the trench by at least 50 cm. The floor should be plastered with mud, with holes of approximately 25 cm in diameter left at 1-metre intervals. (A reinforced concrete slab should be used if possible.) Once the trench is filled to about 30 cm below ground level it should be filled in with earth and a new trench should be dug.

The bore-hole latrine

If the subsoil is not rocky and the water-table is very low (at least 7 m below the ground level), a hole can be made with an earth-auger; it should be about 40 cm in diameter and 5–6 m deep and should not penetrate the water-table. There should be one bore-hole latrine for every 20 people.

Septic tanks

If the soil is sandy or very wet, trench latrines are impractical and septic tanks may have to be provided for drainage. These are normally drained by gravity, which makes it necessary to build an elevated platform for latrines (or to site latrines on suitably sloping terrain). Septic tanks are widely available at relatively low cost; installation should be straightforward but expert advice may be needed. Equipment should be available for desludging the septic tanks regularly.

Washing facilities

Washing is no problem when water supplies are plentiful. When the number of water points is limited, however, providing a special washing facility will save water and make it easier for people to collect. A suitable facility can be constructed on site with available materials (e.g. pierced oil drums for showers). If it is feasible, facilities such as fuel and suitable containers should be provided for boiling clothes. A changing and drying area should be provided for people who have only one set of clothes.

Drainage of surface water from washing facilities and around water collection points should be given proper consideration.

Solid waste disposal

Facilities for the disposal of garbage are an important aspect of environmental sanitation. In a camp situation arrangements should be made for sanitary disposal of domestic wastes around housing units or at an appropriate nearby site; in urban situations, waste should be collected regularly and disposed of at a more distant site. Medical wastes (from hospital, clinics, health centres, etc.) should be managed separately from domestic wastes (by means of incineration or burial in deep pits).

CHAPTER 7

The context: emergency preparedness and response programmes

Community and national preparedness

Recent decades have witnessed droughts, wars, and other disasters on a vast scale. Such events can affect provinces, countries, and groups of countries over periods of months or even years. To take just one example, the United Nations relief programme in Angola assisted 3.3 million people in July 1994, most of whom had been exposed to food shortages and at risk of nutritional deficiencies and starvation for at least 4 years.

These trends point to the need for strategies and operational systems that can:

- detect vulnerability to nutritional deficiencies and address the problem through development programmes;
- prepare contingency plans and monitor early warning indicators;
- activate the plans, and combat nutritional emergencies when they occur;
- ensure that relief efforts facilitate long-term rehabilitation.

As discussed elsewhere in this manual, effective relief hinges upon thorough emergency preparedness, which must be designed according to the nature of the disasters that are prevalent in a given area and integrated within plans and programmes for socioeconomic development.

In countries that are prone to drought or other causes of mass food shortages, preparedness must include a strong food and nutrition component, supported by adequate human and institutional capacities. A consistent investment in relevant training is essential, as well as the development of policies, programmes, contingency plans, systems for surveillance, early warning and buffer stocks; all of these should be linked with general national policies and programmes for health, emergency preparedness, and food security.

Once disaster indicators reach "alert" levels, the wide dissemination of information, the awareness of the public, and the responsiveness of political decision-makers will be the key factors in prompt activation of the response. For an emergency to be "managed" it must first be officially acknowledged.

Planning for nutritional emergencies, as a part of health planning, dovetails into multisectoral emergency planning, is based on the same guiding principles, and uses the same processes. Health professionals, and emergency health planning groups in particular, must be familiar with the multisectoral emergency plans at their level, whether this be community, district, provincial, or national. These plans will inform them of the roles and responsibilities of the other sectors involved (police and investigation, search and rescue, social welfare, agriculture and trade, transport and lifelines, and communications) and the control management structures. Representatives of the health sector should be appointed to multisectoral planning committees at national, provincial, and community levels.

National capacity needs to be developed and maintained to prevent emergencies as far as possible, and to deal with them when they do occur. Annex 9 outlines the educational and training aspects of such capacity development.

Representatives of organizations that lend support to the health ministry (e.g. community organizations such as those representing women or farmers, Red

Cross or Red Crescent, private health sector, specialized institutions, universities, the armed forces) should participate in the planning process. These organizations should also develop their own plans, and determine how they will be coordinated with health and other sectors.

The final health sector plan itself is only one of the results of the planning process, and the capacity and will to implement it fully are essential.

The key to successful emergency preparedness and response is cooperation and coordination across all levels:

- The national emergency health planning committee and the national emergency health manager should cooperate with the national emergency management organization, and provide policy and standards to the health sector at national, provincial, and community levels.
- All health service providers, across all health disciplines, should work together in emergency preparedness and response.
- Health sector planning and response should dovetail with multisectoral planning and response.

Coordination

Widespread food shortages call for large-scale relief programmes as well as policies to deal with the underlying causes. Depending on the magnitude of the crisis, intersectoral committees are generally required at both national and subnational levels. The committees will bring together the national authorities, the international donors, the specialized United Nations agencies, and nongovernmental organizations, in order to:

- define the responsibilities of the participating agencies/individuals, on a sectoral or geographical basis;
- organize the initial rapid assessment of the problem and of the needs;
- adopt appropriate strategies and standard procedures for feeding programmes, ration allocations, supplementation, training, surveillance, and reporting;
- oversee the procurement of food and the mobilization of human, material, and financial resources for the relief programme;
- monitor the delivery and distribution of relief and the evolution of needs and operations;
- monitor stocks and agree on estimates of future food requirements;
- meet regularly and frequently to share all relevant information, and modify plans and strategies as necessary;
- ensure liaison with the media.

It is important that an intersectoral committee has access to technical expertise in the areas of health, nutrition, food security or vulnerability assessment, food safety and control, and logistics. Interdisciplinary and interdepartmental technical committees or mechanisms may need to be established for some of these areas of concern and action at the national level. Such working groups may also be needed at the local level, set up — for instance — by district authorities. Their purpose at both levels is to ensure that vital action is not overlooked, because it is often needed at the interface between habitual areas of action of different ministries or organizations, and also to prevent duplicated, or even contradictory, action by different partners in the emergency response network.

A central logistic support unit will be needed to keep track of in-country procurements, imports, customs clearances, transportation of commodities (at least as far as the district level), warehousing, and position of stocks.

In situations of conflict, which represent complex emergencies, this logistic unit will need specific capacities — for airlifts, escort for convoys, monitoring of accessibility, and security. In addition, special agreements and procedures will be needed for the safe delivery of humanitarian assistance, e.g. clearance of convoys and airlifts, combat-free humanitarian corridors, predetermined cease-fire periods.

In terms of overall authority and coordination, the arrangements vary:

- Sometimes, national management bodies for emergency preparedness and response are already in place, normally in the presidential or prime ministerial office.
- A special relief/rehabilitation commission is sometimes established, under the auspices of a specialized ministry; such bodies may even organize their own health services, although this is not a desirable arrangement.
- A technical ministry or a specialized agency may be given lead responsibility, largely on the basis of its statutory role (e.g. planning or finance) or of its capacities at field level (e.g. agriculture, local government, grain marketing authority).
- To ensure the neutrality of humanitarian assistance in complex emergencies, a special United Nations coordinating office is sometimes established, under the authority of a Special Representative of the UN Secretary General whose responsibility is to guarantee the political aspects of the arrangement.

Whatever the setting, the intersectoral committee will ordinarily include representatives from the ministries of (or responsible for) planning, finance, the interior, local government, health, social welfare, transport, agriculture, trade, environment, communications, and civil protection. The police and armed forces can usually deploy considerable logistic capacities and should also be involved. Liaison with the armed forces is an absolute necessity when security considerations prevail, such as in complex emergencies.

The capacity of the ministry of health to play its full role in the committee(s) — providing nutritional and epidemiological updates, technical guidance on the scope of general and selective feeding programmes, advice on micronutrient supplementation, information on disease control activities, etc. — is an essential component of emergency preparedness.

Apart from funds for the procurement of relief food, financial arrangements have to be made to cover the costs of transport and warehousing, nutritional surveillance, communications, complementary activities in fields such as water and health, and general programme overheads. Financial resources have to be mobilized either from the state budget or from regular aid programmes; failing this, extraordinary arrangements have to be made with governments, NGOs, or international donors. This process will be coordinated by the intersectoral committee, often in liaison with the UN Department of Humanitarian Affairs, relevant UN agencies, and bilateral organizations, at the national, regional, or agency headquarters level.

These administrative, technical, and financial mechanisms take time to establish and implement; during this lead-time the emergency is likely to grow in magnitude and gravity. If lines of authority, responsibilities, administrative arrangements, contingency funds, and procedures for their activation are previously agreed as part of a national preparedness plan, and made known to all involved, precious time will be saved.

Steps in this direction have been taken by recent UN initiatives, in which WHO participates, such as the country Disaster Management Team (DMT) and the Disaster Management Training Programme (UNDMTP).

Operations

Within the overall objectives of reducing the suffering of the community and facilitating the resumption of production and development, the operations should adhere to a set of strategic criteria:

- fostering community participation in management and ownership of programmes, and local capacity-building;
- containing the displacement of the population;
- optimizing food aid;
- minimizing dependency and facilitating rehabilitation.

Fostering ownership, participation, and capacities

Coordinating mechanisms are needed at subnational as well as national level. If a vast area is affected, it is usually necessary, through the ministry of local government, to establish intersectoral committees at provincial/regional level and on down, to village, or at least district/municipal, level. There, according to the circumstances, the leading role may be played by whichever ministry, department, or even local NGO, has the greatest capacities — although the intersectoral character of the exercise must be safeguarded.

These committees must include representatives of the beneficiaries, at least at district level where relief and rehabilitation are more directly linked with development. The national relief strategy should make effective provisions for the involvement of local and traditional leaders and civil organizations, including religious groupings, women's groups, and NGOs. This applies whether the affected population is located in cities, villages, or camps. National/local ownership and participation will also be strengthened if the international agencies involved recruit local personnel for their programmes of emergency assistance.

National guidelines and plans will have to be adapted locally. The selection of the beneficiaries of food-aid will imply study, dialogue with affected communities, and decisions — inevitably difficult — on the part of the authorities. Technical criteria from the central level (e.g. clear guidelines on nutrition from the ministry of health) will help in targeting the most vulnerable, in monitoring their needs, and in substantiating administrative decisions that affect the community.

Local arrangements for the distribution of relief may include:

- food cards or stamps, ration shops, cash-for-work, cash-for-food projects, food-for-work programmes, which will ensure the general ration;
- supplementary feeding for children under 5 years old, pregnant women and possibly lactating women, the chronically ill, the elderly, children in primary schools.

The actual distribution of food will need direct support activities, including monitoring the situation and the impact of relief through anthropometric and socio-economic surveys, identifying local projects, and improving vital infrastructures (wells, roads, bridges, warehouses, etc.). Therapeutic feeding in cases of severe malnutrition should be integrated in wider programmes of emergency response implemented and coordinated by the district health team, often in collaboration with national and international NGOs.

Transparency and accountability in the management of relief will usually have a positive influence on the mobilization of resources: in a nationwide emergency, targeting of aid is generally based not only on the numbers of people in need but also on local management capacities. Any records that the district authorities are able to keep of the operations will be useful once the crisis is over. The lessons learnt will help in modifying the preparedness and development plans of the district, and addressing vulnerabilities and hazards in the medium and long term.

Substantial administrative and logistic capacity can be drawn from line ministries and departments, as well as from individual volunteers, local NGOs, religious groups, etc., but much training will be required. Again, identifying resources, distributing tasks, and conducting training all take time, and would be best undertaken as part of district preparedness programmes, before an emergency occurs. In famine-prone areas, all rural development activities should include a preparedness component; health and nutrition education projects should include guidance on surviving bad years, as well as on improving nutritional status in good years.

Nevertheless, if efforts to build capacity have not been made in advance of an emergency, they will have to be made during the relief and rehabilitation phases; adequate resources must be made available for this in the framework of the relief programme.

Containing the displacement of the population

The more widespread is the food distribution system, the less people will be forced to move away from their homes. Containment of displacement — and of potentially hazardous concentrations of beneficiaries — is an important yardstick of the success of a relief programme. All efforts should be made to reach the affected people, and minister to their needs, wherever they are. Clear information on the criteria of eligibility for relief and on the places, modes, and timetables of distribution must be disseminated, and strict adherence to schedules and procedures is essential.

In the early stages of a crisis, or at least as long as local market systems continue to function, cash-for-food projects can enable vulnerable households to buy food, plus farm tools and seeds for the next season's crop. In this way, families enter the local credit market and do not need to migrate. Food-for-work projects are also effective in holding families and the communities together, by providing food security (abeit temporary, dependent, and unsustainable) and a social framework of shared occupations and objectives.

Use can be made of existing government, communal, or private commercial networks to ensure the most viable, widespread system for the distribution of food. Relief distribution centres can be set up in rural markets or at government marketing outlets, and be supplied from the provincial or regional capital. Private transporters and NGOs can assist with logistics.

Concentrating affected people in refugee or displaced-person camps is not desirable and should be contemplated only as a last resort. It may be a typical solution in conflict situations, when beneficiaries need to be in secure and accessible areas, but camps entail a number of risks and problems including the following:

- Overcrowding and generally poor living conditions, restricted access to water, and limited sanitation contribute to the creation of new and specific health hazards.
- Farming land may be too far away, too scarce, or unsuitable for production.
- Prolonged use of non-traditional foods (e.g. milled cereal flour, instead of grains) can lead to difficulties in returning to traditional lifestyles later.
- Too many decisions made by outsiders cause loss of initiative and of community leadership, and may even lead to mental depression; dependency may become so entrenched that dispersing camps is difficult, even when the emergency has ended.
- Normal social patterns are disrupted, so that traditional "safety nets" and coping mechanisms are damaged. New, untested power structures can emerge, and disputes may arise with host populations or among displaced groups with diverse political or ethnic affiliations.
- Camps may become security liabilities, particularly if they are large. Large camps are difficult to manage, and faulty management can lead to internal tensions and even riots. In low-intensity conflicts, camps can become political targets and may be attacked or infiltrated by the combatants.

Optimizing food aid

As far as possible, food and other relief items should be procured within the country by purchasing and transporting surpluses from unaffected areas. This reduces the programme's overhead costs, and partially compensates for the losses caused to the country's economy by the disaster.

Relief operations are expensive to mount and lose cost-effectiveness if the rations that are distributed have inadequate caloric value or if food aid is spread too thinly. A balanced food-basket should be a concern in the economy of the programme: if the distribution of the different foods is not well coordinated, for instance, beneficiaries may have to survive for considerable periods on only one food item, perhaps drawing all their energy requirements from pulses rather than primarily from cereals.

Adequate health resources and activities at community and district levels are key factors in both offsetting the increased vulnerability and ensuring that the beneficiaries profit fully from the food that they receive. Besides the surveys and supplementary and therapeutic feeding programmes, comprehensive intersectoral activities for the control of communicable diseases will also be a priority as mentioned above. Special strategies and procedures will be needed if the district health team is to liaise effectively with other sectors, coordinate with national and international NGOs that may be new in the area, and adapt to the emergency needs.

Intensified health education and, when possible, outreach activities should be instituted to compensate for disruptions in the community's participation in immunizations, mother and child health, etc. Mothers can often be reached where they queue for food or water or when they enrol in food-for-work schemes.

Special training and foodstuffs may be needed, in the field and in referral hospitals, for the diagnosis and management of acute malnutrition and micronutrient deficiencies (see Chapters 2 and 5).

In complex emergencies, and in all situations involving mass movements and concentrations of people, the district health team will need special capacities — such as guidelines, resources, and back-up from the provincial level — in order to assist refugees or displaced populations in temporary shelters and camps. The team must ensure that:

- health considerations and technical guidelines are reflected in all intersectoral decisions concerning site-planning, length of stay, food, water, shelter, sanitation, special care for vulnerable groups, etc;
- people undergo health and nutritional screening on arrival;
- in transit or after arrival in a camp, people have access to primary health care facilities and are adequately covered by disease surveillance and control activities.

The vulnerabilities and needs of the health sector itself should also be addressed. During a drought, some health units may lack water; hospitals will then have to make special provisions for the feeding of inpatients and staff, and for maintaining cleanliness. Health personnel, especially community workers, will suffer from the food shortages and the economic crisis, just like the rest of the population: they may leave, or at least lose their motivation for work. Special incentives and alternative solutions, e.g. food-for-work schemes, may be needed for them.

At times, certain positive features will arise from an emergency situation. For instance, the surveys and the selective feeding programmes can provide opportunities for strengthening mother and child health programmes and for introducing nutritional surveillance routines that can continue after the emergency. The district health team will need additional training, strong supervision, administrative and logistic support, and encouragement from the provincial and national levels. The responsibilities and the tasks of the entire health sector will increase, from the grassroots up to the national level. In particular, there will be greater demand for information and services. Coordination with the other sectors and external partners will also represent an additional workload, to be carried often under pressure and in generally difficult conditions. Plans for emergency relief should therefore always provide for adequate institutional strengthening at all levels.

Psychosocial and mental health concerns

The dislocations associated with emergencies affect psychological and social health, sometimes to an extreme extent. Relief efforts need to contribute to the maintenance of self-esteem and resilience in individuals, families, and communities; restoring their ability to cope and to take control of their lives is a reason for involving them in relief activities and organization. Efforts may be needed to retain the cohesion of families and groups, or even to facilitate new groupings and a new social fabric, by means such as self-help groups, informal adoptions, joint food preparation, etc. Social groups obliged to modify their way of life may need help and confidence-building measures while they learn new technologies and, often, modify their aspirations (for example, when nomads have to become small traders). Children caught up in an emergency are particularly vulnerable to mental scarring and babies to poor cognitive and psychosocial development. Every effort must be made to keep infants and children with their mothers, to promote continuing breast-feeding, and to maintain and strengthen loving care within the family (helped, for example, by preparing food and eating together as a unit).

Minimizing dependency and facilitating rehabilitation

Relief should aim to minimize dependency on the part of the beneficiaries and to facilitate rehabilitation and development. The relief plan, as well as the actual operations, should put as much emphasis on encouraging the beneficiaries in efforts to resume production and achieve future food security, as on distributing food. Food aid can thus be a versatile tool: with international understanding and the support of a national policy framework, and through creative programmes and projects, it can do more than simply ensuring the short-term survival of the population.

In some countries, preparedness plans allow for the prompt creation of employment through development or rehabilitation programmes, instituted on a cash-for-work basis. As noted above, cash-for-food projects at community level can promote self-reliance, ensure access to food and farming inputs, and inject cash into the local economy. Cash-for-food schemes can also be linked to rehabilitation and development activities. "Programme" food aid of this sort is usually in the form of cereals which are sold at the national level (particularly in cities); the proceeds of sale are used by government to support development activities at the appropriate local level. Great care should be exercised to ensure that this food does not, by undercutting local market prices, impoverish local farmers and shopkeepers.

Food-for-work schemes are often typical features of emergency relief programmes. On a large scale, they are usually directed to improving infrastructure. In the short term, for instance, roads and bridges may be rebuilt or improved to facilitate distribution of food; in the medium and long term, goals include rehabilitation, food security, and development (e.g. wells, irrigation, drainage schemes, terracing, tree planting, construction of health posts and schools). Recently — and with technical supervision — food-for-work schemes have also been used for mine-clearance programmes in post-conflict situations.

On a smaller scale, food-for-work can support a wide range of activities, particularly through NGO projects, for production, income-generation, community services, and vocational training. Some experience, however, seems to indicate that enrollment of mothers in food-for-work programmes may have a negative impact on the health of their children, and these programmes should therefore provide at least supplementary feeding for children under 5 years old and should always support breast-feeding.

For some categories of beneficiaries, e.g. refugees, food aid represents the only sort of income and their only support on the road to self-reliance. Many researchers therefore believe that governments and relief agencies should demonstrate greater flexibility vis-à-vis the sale of relief food, provided that this does not affect local production and markets.

If relocation is absolutely necessary — and acceptable — the beneficiaries should be moved into areas that can provide good conditions in terms of shelter, water, and environment (e.g. areas that are free of disease vectors). It should also be possible for agricultural production to be successfully resumed, and so there must be suitable land, seeds and tools must be available, and access to markets, for the sale of surplus production, should be good.

Various other aspects of resettlement should be considered in order to avoid potential conflicts between the host population and newcomers:

- Programmes will be needed to reduce the strain of the incoming population on the capacity of the resettlement area. Roads and bridges, wells, clinics, and schools may have to be built; special measures may be needed to avoid the destruction of trees or other vegetation, and to ensure soil and water conservation. Again, food-for-work or cash-for-work schemes may be useful in this.
- The host communities should be involved in the decisions concerning the resettlement; significant human and material support may have to be provided.
- To minimize the danger of competition for scarce resources, countries that are vulnerable to large population movements (e.g. those that share borders with countries at war, or those that are prone to drought) should make appropriate provisions in their development and preparedness plans, identifying in advance locations that may be suitable for temporary settlements or for resettlement schemes.

Administration of distribution centres and camps

All those responsible for management should be of sound and strong enough character to withstand the pressures that may come from the beneficiaries, from external organizations, or from both. They should also be thoroughly familiar with the language and culture of the beneficiaries and with the geography of the area.

The following categories of personnel will be needed on site:

- supervisors (for food distribution and for water and sanitation facilities);
- registry clerks (and possibly assistants, depending on the size of the operation);
- store-keepers and food supervisors trained in food safety;
- guards for food stocks (security may be provided by the government).

Hired staff should live close to the place of work. Personnel needed for food distribution, cooking, and other support tasks should be recruited from among the beneficiaries on a clearly defined cash- or food-for-work basis.

An office will be needed, with the following equipment:

- registry books;
- a map of the area or camp, showing the different sectors and facilities;
- a chart or a blackboard, indicating the number of inhabitants in each sector;
- a clear and complete list of all personnel.

The office should have a sheltered porch for waiting visitors, and should always be locked after working hours.

Setting up a committee of representatives of the beneficiaries will help in securing the community's full participation in the programme. If there is no formal committee, there should be at least a contact group consisting of one person from each sector of the community. This committee/contact group can hold discussions with the responsible officers about food distribution and other important events (immunization schedules, changes in the programmes, official visits, etc.). It will also be responsible for improving the living conditions in the community, including development of primary health care and related facilities, services, and activities for agriculture and education.

These initiatives are especially important in refugee and displaced-person camps, where there are more pressing needs and greater opportunities for promoting safe water supplies, sanitation, immunizations, literacy, special care for the vulnerable, women's groups, income-generating activities, etc.

Logistics

Transportation

Transportation of foodstuffs — which are bulky — is often the cause of bottlenecks and delays in relief operations. Considerations include the following:

- Transporting the full dry ration (36 000 kg) for 1 week for 10 000 people requires 12 3-ton trucks.
- A jeep or a minibus can carry about 500 kg of food, plus a small team of personnel for food distribution and surveillance; 500 kg represent the daily general

ration for 1000 people (200 families) or the supplementary ration for 5500 children.

- Transportation is also needed for supervisory personnel on a full-time basis.
- In bad weather conditions, at least one out of every 10 vehicles will be immobilized at any given time, for maintenance or repair.
- Delays due to bad weather, poor roads, and vehicle breakdown are common.

Storage

All foods are subject to degradation during storage, but some degenerate faster than others and no special measures are taken to preserve perishable foods (vegetables, fruits, animal products). In emergencies, the bulk of the energy requirement is supplied by cereals, and sometimes by pulses and oilseeds. These are usually supplied as dry grain or flour. Grain is more stable than flour because the latter absorbs moisture more rapidly, which favours the multiplication of insects, fungi, and bacteria. Chemical degradation (e.g. rancidity in vegetable oils) may also be a problem.

Careful storage and handling can minimize the waste, and the following rules should be followed:

- The store should have a good roof and should be dry, well ventilated, and as cool as possible. Using modern buildings as warehouses minimizes the problem of rodents, insects, etc. by making access more difficult.
- Products should be kept at least 40 cm off the walls and 10 cm off the floor; bags must lie on pallets, boards, heavy branches, bricks, or a layer of clean dry polyethylene bags or tarpaulins — not directly on the floor.
- Damaged bags must be kept apart from the undamaged (possibly in a separate area); a reserve of good empty bags should be kept so that goods from damaged bags can be repacked.
- Bags should be stacked two by two (i.e. two bags in one direction, then two more on top at 90° to the first two) to allow ventilation; they will also be more stable and easier to count.
- Stacks should be no higher than 2 m; this makes handling easier and reduces the risk of stacks falling.
- Each product should be stored separately and have its own stock card.
- Access to the warehouse should be limited to a few authorized individuals.
- The store must have a lock and the storekeeper should always keep the key and be responsible for it.
- The balance on the stock cards should be checked periodically by counting the actual number of items in the store.
- Stocks should be rotated on the basis of first-in-first-out; new deliveries should not be stacked on top or in front of old stock. Old stocks should be issued before new supplies.

- Labourers should be trained and supervised; this will reduce damage resulting from careless handling.

In bags, 1 tonne (2205 lb or 1000 kg) of cereals or processed food occupies approximately $2\,m^3$; thus 1 tonne of grain stacked 2 m high occupies $1\,m^2$ of floor space. Since space must be left for ventilation and aisles for access, only about 80% of the total floor area of a warehouse is usable for storage. For bulk food supplies, the calculation is as follows:

For 30 000 people using 400 g of grain per person per day for 60 days: $30\,000 \times 400 \times 60 = 720\,000\,000\,g = 720$ tonnes. The volume of this grain is $1440\,m^3$; stacked 2 m high this requires a surface area of $720\,m^2$ + 20% for access and ventilation = $864\,m^2$. A building of $43\,m \times 20\,m$ would provide $860\,m^2$, and one of $50\,m \times 18\,m$ would provide $900\,m^2$.

Further information on food storage may be found in the following publication:

- Walker DJ, ed. *Food storage manual.* Rome, and Chatham, England, World Food Programme and Natural Resources Institute, 1992.

Rats and vermin

Spilled foods and refuse attract rodents, insects, and birds. The best method of control is to keep the food store clean. Broken bags should be stored in a separate area, and the contents should be enclosed in polyethylene bags. Poison baits are not effective in controlling pests.

Fumigation with methyl bromide or phosphine is inexpensive and kills rodents and insects in the store and insects in the bags. However, it is toxic to humans and must be carried out only by trained personnel. If the manufacturer's instructions are carefully followed, fumigation is safe and the food will not be impaired.

Spraying the store regularly with suitable insecticide is also an effective measure, but expert advice must be sought. All bags must be closed and the food protected from direct contact with the insecticide.

Cereals and dried fish are particularly prone to infestation, especially in tropical climates. Infested foods do not lose nutritional value and their safety may not be affected. Wet bags should be dried in the sun before being stored; infested bags should be taken outside and weevils sieved out. Infested cereals or blends should be distributed as soon as possible; weevils and worms will float to the top when the grains are soaked in water. Hard lumps in milk bags are harmless, provided that there is no rancid smell. Foodstuff on which rodents or cats have urinated or defecated can transmit salmonellosis, Lassa fever, or leptospirosis.

ANNEX 1

Nutritional requirements

This annex contains a number of tables that indicate the nutritional requirements (for energy, protein, and micronutrients) for different age and sex groups and overall figures for whole populations with typical demographic and anthropometric profiles of developing countries and industrialized countries.

The complete list of tables is as follows:

Table A1.1 *Energy requirements for emergency-affected populations: developing country profile (demography and anthropometry)*[a,b]

Age (years)	Male[c]		Female[c]		Male + female[c]	
	% of total population	Energy requirement ($kcal_{th}$)	% of total population	Energy requirement ($kcal_{th}$)	% of total population	Energy requirement ($kcal_{th}$)
0	1.31	850	1.27	780	2.59	820
1[d]	1.26	1250	1.20	1190	2.46	1220
2[d]	1.25	1430	1.20	1330	2.45	1380
3[d]	1.25	1560	1.19	1440	2.44	1500
4[d]	1.24	1690	1.19	1540	2.43	1620
0–4	6.32	1320	6.05	1250	12.37	1290
5–9	6.00	1980	5.69	1730	11.69	1860
10–14	5.39	2370	5.13	2040	10.53	2210
15–19	4.89	2700	4.64	2120	9.54	2420
20–59[e]	24.80	2460	23.82	1990	48.63	2230
≥60[e]	3.42	2010	3.82	1780	7.24	1890
Pregnant			2.40	285 (extra)	2.40	285 (extra)
Lactating			2.60	500 (extra)	2.60	500 (extra)
Whole population	50.84	2250	49.16	1910		2080

[a] Energy requirements derived from: *Energy and protein requirements. Report of a Joint FAO/WHO/UNU Expert Consultation.* Geneva, World Health Organization, 1985 (Technical Report Series, No. 724).
Population data (for mid-1995) from United Nations Population Division.

[b] The requirements shown in this table do not take account of the varying fibre content, digestibility, and complex-carbohydrate composition of the diet. In developing countries, the diet usually contains a relatively high proportion of fibre and less-available carbohydrate. The carbohydrate content of foods may be expressed in terms of its various components (starches, sugars, fibre, cellulose, lignins, etc.) or simply as the calculated "difference" between total weight and the sum of other components (fat, protein, minerals, and water). If the Atwater factor ($4\,kcal_{th}/g$) is applied to carbohydrate by difference, the real energy available in the food should be reduced by 5%, i.e. the "requirement" for this type of diet should be increased by 5%. Thus the energy requirement indicated in this table for the whole population (men, women, and both combined) should be increased by $100\,kcal_{th}$. The correction factor is not applicable if the energy content of food is expressed in terms of true available energy.

[c] Adult weight: males 60 kg, females 52 kg.

[d] Population estimates for years 1, 2, 3, and 4 are not available from the United Nations; estimates were therefore made by interpolation from the UN data for 0 and 5 years.

[e] Basal metabolic rate (BMR) is the rate of energy expenditure of the body when at complete rest (e.g. during sleep); the figures given here for energy requirements are for "light" activity levels (1.55 × BMR for males, 1.56 × BMR for females). For adjustments for moderate and heavy activity, see Table A1.3.

Table A1.2 *Energy requirements for emergency-affected populations: industrialized country profile (demography and anthropometry)*[a,b]

Age (years)	Male[c]		Female[c]		Male + female[c]	
	% of total population	Energy requirement ($kcal_{th}$)	% of total population	Energy requirement ($kcal_{th}$)	% of total population	Energy requirement ($kcal_{th}$)
0	0.62	800	0.59	740	1.22	820
1[d]	0.62	1200	0.60	1140	1.22	1220
2[d]	0.63	1410	0.60	1310	1.22	1380
3[d]	0.63	1560	0.60	1440	1.23	1500
4[d]	0.65	1690	0.62	1540	1.27	1620
0–4	3.16	1330	3.00	1240	6.16	1290
5–9	3.42	1980	3.26	1760	6.67	1860
10–14	3.48	2390	3.33	2050	6.81	2210
15–19	3.49	2780	3.34	2160	6.83	2420
20–59[e]	27.56	2590	27.68	2090	55.24	2230
≥60[e]	7.44	2160	10.84	1880	18.28	1890
Pregnant			1.2	200 (extra)	1.2	200 (extra)
Lactating			0.3	500 (extra)	0.3	500 (extra)
Whole population	48.55	2400	51.45	1980		2180

[a] Energy requirements derived from: *Energy and protein requirements. Report of a Joint FAO/WHO/UNU Expert Consultation.* Geneva, World Health Organization, 1985 (Technical Report Series, No. 724).
Population data (for mid-1995) from United Nations Population Division.

[b] The requirements shown in this table do not take account of the varying fibre content, digestibility, and complex-carbohydrate composition of the diet. In industrialized countries, the diet usually contains a relatively lower proportion of fibre than in developing countries. The carbohydrate content of foods may be expressed in terms of its various components (starches, sugars, fibre, cellulose, lignins, etc.) or simply as the calculated "difference" between total weight and the sum of other components (fat, protein, minerals, and water). If the Atwater factor ($4\,kcal_{th}/g$) is applied to carbohydrate by difference, the real energy available in the food should be reduced by 2.5%, i.e. the "requirement" for this type of diet should be increased by 2.5%. Thus the energy requirement indicated in this table for the whole population (men, women, and both combined) should be increased by $50\,kcal_{th}$. The correction factor is not applicable if the energy content of food is expressed in terms of true available energy.

[c] Adult weight: males 67 kg, females 55 kg.

[d] Population estimates for years 1, 2, 3, and 4 are not available from the United Nations; estimates were therefore made by interpolation from the UN data for 0 and 5 years.

[e] Basal metabolic rate (BMR) is the rate of energy expenditure of the body when at complete rest (e.g. during sleep); the figures given here for energy requirements are for "light" activity levels (1.55 × BMR for males, 1.56 × BMR for females). For adjustments for moderate and heavy activity, see Table A1.3.

Table A1.3 *Mean energy requirements and recommended adjustments for different activity levels, environmental temperatures, and food losses during transport*[a]

	Developing country	Industrialized country
Mean energy requirement ($kcal_{th}$)	**2080**	**2180**
Adjustment to energy requirement ($kcal_{th}$) for activity level:		
Moderate[b]		
Adult[c] males	+360	+370
Adult[c] females	+100	+105
Whole population (adults + children)	+140	+180
Heavy[b]		
Adult[c] males	+850	+890
Adult[c] females	+330	+340
Whole population	+350	+460
Adjustment to energy requirement ($kcal_{th}$) for mean daily temperature:		
20 °C	—	
15 °C	+100	
10 °C	+200	
5 °C	+300	
0 °C	+400	
Adjustment to energy requirement ($kcal_{th}$) for food losses in transport:		
Country with port	+5%	
Landlocked country	+10%	

[a] Data derived from: *Energy and protein requirements. Report of a Joint FAO/WHO/UNU Expert Consultation.* Geneva, World Health Organization, 1985 (Technical Report Series, No. 724).

[b] Energy requirements for moderate activity are calculated as 1.78 × BMR for males and 1.64 × BMR for females, and for heavy activity as 2.10 × BMR for males and 1.82 × BMR for females.

[c] Age ≥18 years.

Table A1.4 *Protein requirements: developing country profile*[a]

Age (years)	Male[b]			Female[b]			Male and female[b]		
	% of total population	Reference protein[c] (g/day)	Mixed cereal/pulse diet[d] (g/day)	% of total population	Reference protein[c] (g/day)	Mixed cereal/pulse diet[d] (g/day)	% of total population	Reference protein[c] (g/day)	Mixed cereal/pulse diet[d] (g/day)
0	1.31	12.9	12.9[e]	1.27	11.9	11.9[e]	2.59	12.4	12.4[e]
1[f]	1.26	14.1	23.7	1.20	13.3	22.3	2.46	13.7	23.0
2[f]	1.25	15.5	26.2	1.20	15.0	25.2	2.45	15.2	25.5
3[f]	1.25	16.9	28.4	1.19	16.5	27.7	2.44	16.7	28.1
4[f]	1.24	18.5	31.1	1.19	17.3	29.1	2.43	17.9	30.1
0–4	6.32	15.6	26.2	6.05	14.7	24.7	12.37	15.2	25.5
5–9	6.00	24.3	33.3	5.69	23.9	32.7	11.69	24.1	33.0
10–14	5.39	39.0	49.1	5.13	40.4	50.9	10.53	39.7	50.0
15–19	4.89	52.2	61.6	4.64	43.8	51.7	9.54	48.0	56.6
20–59	24.80	45.0	53.1	23.82	39.0	46.0	48.63	42.0	49.6
60+	3.42	45.0	53.1	3.82	39.0	46.0	7.24	42.0	49.6
Pregnant				2.4	6.0 (extra)	7.1 (extra)	2.4	6.0 (extra)	7.1 (extra)
Lactating:									
1st 6 m				1.0	16.0 (extra)	18.9 (extra)	1.0	16.0 (extra)	18.9 (extra)
2nd 6 m				0.8	12.0 (extra)	14.2 (extra)	0.8	12.0 (extra)	14.2 (extra)
over 12 m				0.8	11.0 (extra)	13.0 (extra)	0.8	11.0 (extra)	13.0 (extra)
Whole population	50.84	39.0	47.8	49.16	35.2	43.2		37.1	45.6

[a] Requirements derived from: *Energy and protein requirements. Report of a Joint FAO/WHO/UNU Expert Consultation.* Geneva, World Health Organization, 1985 (Technical Report Series, No. 724).

[b] Adult weight: males 60 kg, females 52 kg.

[c] Reference protein is protein with the quality and digestibility of milk or egg.

[d] Mixed cereal/pulse diet includes cereals, pulses, and vegetables as, for instance, in the rural Tunisian diet.

[e] Assuming fully breast-fed.

[f] Population estimates for years 1, 2, 3, and 4 are not available from the United Nations; estimates were therefore made by interpolation from the UN data for 0 and 5 years.

Table A1.5 *Protein requirements: industrialized country profile*[a]

Age (years)	Male[b]			Female[b]			Male and female[b]		
	% of total population	Reference protein[c] (g/day)	Mixed cereal/pulse diet[d] (g/day)	% of total population	Reference protein[c] (g/day)	Mixed cereal/pulse diet[d] (g/day)	% of total population	Reference protein[c] (g/day)	Mixed cereal/pulse diet[d] (g/day)
0	0.62	12.9	21.7[e]	0.59	11.9	20.0[e]	1.22	12.3	20.7[e]
1[f]	0.62	14.1	23.7	0.60	13.3	22.3	1.22	14.0	23.5
2[f]	0.63	15.5	26.0	0.60	15.0	25.2	1.22	15.5	25.9
3[f]	0.63	16.9	28.4	0.60	16.5	27.7	1.23	16.7	28.1
4[f]	0.65	18.5	31.1	0.62	17.3	28.6	1.27	17.9	30.1
0–4	3.16	15.7	26.1	3.00	14.9	25.0	6.16	15.3	25.6
5–9	3.42	24.4	33.4	3.26	24.1	33.0	6.67	24.3	40.6
10–14	3.48	42.1	53.0	3.33	41.5	52.3	6.81	41.8	52.7
15–19	3.49	54.4	64.2	3.34	44.7	52.7	6.83	49.7	58.6
20–59	27.56	50.2	59.2	27.68	41.2	48.6	55.24	45.9	54.2
60+	7.44	50.2	59.2	10.84	41.2	48.68	18.28	44.9	53.0
Pregnant				1.2	6.0 (extra)	7.1 (extra)	1.2	6.0 (extra)	7.1 (extra)
Lactating:									
1st 6 m				0.2[e]	16.0 (extra)	18.9 (extra)	0.2[e]	16.0 (extra)	18.9 (extra)
2nd 6 m				0.1	12.0 (extra)	14.2 (extra)	0.1	12.0 (extra)	14.2 (extra)
Whole population	48.55	45.9	55.1	51.45	39.5	53.9		42.4	54.4

[a] Requirements derived from: *Energy and protein requirements. Report of a Joint FAO/WHO/UNU Expert Consultation.* Geneva, World Health Organization, 1985 (Technical Report Series, No. 724).

[b] Adult weight: males 67 kg, females 55 kg.

[c] Reference protein is protein with the quality and digestibility of milk or egg.

[d] Mixed cereal/pulse diet includes cereals, pulses, and vegetables as, for instance, in the rural Tunisian diet.

[e] Assuming 3 months of breast-feeding.

[f] Population estimates for years 1, 2, 3, and 4 are not available from the United Nations; estimates were therefore made by interpolation from the UN data for 0 and 5 years.

***Table A1.6** Vitamin requirements (safe levels of intake): developing and industrialized countries*[a]

Age (years)	Vitamin A[b] (μg retinol)	Vitamin D[c] (μg calciferol)	Thiamine[d,e] (mg)	Riboflavin[d,e] (mg)	Niacin equivalents[d,e] (mg)	Folic acid[b] (μg)	Vitamin B_{12}[b] (μg)	Ascorbic acid (mg)
0	350	10.0	0.3	0.5	4.2	24	0.1	20
1	400	10.0	0.5	0.8	6.4	50	0.45	20
2	400	10.0	0.55	0.9	7.5	50	0.53	20
3	400	10.0	0.60	1.0	8.2	50	0.61	20
4	400	10.0	0.65	1.1	8.9	50	0.69	20
0–4	390	10.0	0.5	0.8	7.1	45	0.50	20
5–9	400	2.5	0.75	1.2	10.3	80	0.82	20
10–14 M	550	2.5	0.95	1.6	13.1	150	1.0	25
10–14 F	550	2.5	0.8	1.35	11.3	130	1.0	25
10–14 M+F	550	2.5	0.9	1.5	12.2	140	1.0	25
15–19 M	600	2.5	1.1	1.8	15.3	200	1.0	30
15–19 F	500	2.5	0.9	1.4	11.9	170	1.0	30
15–19 M+F	550	2.5	1.0	1.6	13.6	185	1.0	30
20–59 M	600	2.5	1.0	1.7	14.5	200	1.0	30
20–59 F	500	2.5	0.8	1.4	11.5	170	1.0	30
20–59 M+F	570	2.5	0.9	1.55	12.9	185	1.0	30
60+ M	600	3.2	0.9	1.4	11.9	200	1.0	30
60+ F	500	3.2	0.75	1.2	10.3	170	1.0	30
60+ M+F	540	3.2	0.8	1.3	10.9	185	1.0	30
Pregnant	100 (extra)	7.5 (extra)	0.1 (extra)	0.1 (extra)	1.1 (extra)	250 (extra)	0.4 (extra)	20 (extra)
Lactating	350 (extra)	7.5 (extra)	0.2 (extra)	0.3 (extra)	2.7 (extra)	100 (extra)	0.3 (extra)	20 (extra)
Whole population	500	3.2–3.8[f]	0.9	1.4	12.0	160	0.9	28

[a] Based on Table 1 of Passmore R et al. *Handbook on human nutritional requirements.* Geneva, World Health Organization, 1974 (WHO Monograph Series, No. 61).

[b] Data derived from: *Requirements of vitamin A, iron, folate and vitamin B12. Report of a Joint FAO/WHO Expert Consultation.* Rome, Food and Agriculture Organization of the United Nations, 1985 (FAO Food and Nutrition Series, No. 23).

[c] Data derived from: *Requirements of ascorbic acid, vitamin D, vitamin B12, folate and iron, Report of a Joint FAO/WHO Expert Group.* Geneva, World Health Organization, 1970 (WHO Technical Report Series, No. 470), and Rome, Food and Agriculture Organization of the United Nations, 1970 (FAO Nutrition Meetings Report Series, No. 47).

[d] Data derived from: *Requirements of vitamin A, thiamine, riboflavine and niacin. Report of a Joint FAO/WHO Expert Group.* Geneva, World Health Organization, 1967 (WHO Technical Report Series No. 362), and Rome, Food and Agriculture Organization of the United Nations, 1965 (FAO Food and Nutrition Series, No. 8).

[e] B vitamin requirements are proportional to energy intake and are calculated as follows:
thiamine: 0.4 mg per 1000 $kcal_{th}$ ingested
riboflavin: 0.6 mg per 1000 $kcal_{th}$ ingested
niacin equivalents: 6.6 mg per 1000 $kcal_{th}$ ingested

[f] The higher figure is for developing countries because of the larger proportion of children under 5 years whose requirement is greater.

Table A1.7 *Daily dietary mineral requirements (safe levels of intake): developing and industrialized countries*[a]

Age (years)	Calcium[b] (g)	Iron (mg), bioavailability:[c]				Iodine[d] (μg)
		very low (<5%)	low (5–9%)	moderate (10–18%)	high (>19%)	
0	0.5–0.6	24	13	6	4	50–90
1	0.4–0.5	15	8	4	3	90
2	0.4–0.5	16	8	4	3	90
3	0.4–0.5	17	9	5	3	90
4	0.4–0.5	18	9	5	3	90
0–4	0.4–0.5	18	9	5	3	90
5–9	0.4–0.5	29	16	8	4	110
10–14 M	0.6–0.7	45	24	12	7	140
10–14 F	0.6–0.7	50	27	13	8	140
10–14 M+F	0.6–0.7	47	26	12.5	7.5	140
15–19 M	0.5–0.6	28	15	10	7	150
15–19 F	0.5–0.6	60	32	16	10	150
15–19 M+F	0.5–0.6	44	24	12	8.5	150
20–59 M	0.4–0.5	28	15	8	5	150
20–59 F	0.4–0.5	59	32	16	11	150
20–59 M+F	0.4–0.5	43	23	12	8	150
60+	0.4–0.5	26	15	7	4.5	150
Pregnant (latter half)	0.6–0.7 (extra)	120–240[e] (extra)	60–120[e] (extra)	30–60[e] (extra)	20–50[e] (extra)	50 (extra)
Lactating (first 6 m)	0.6–0.7 (extra)	33	17	9	6	50 (extra)
Postmenopausal	0.4–0.5	26	15	6	4	150
Whole population	0.45–0.55	41	22	11	7	150

[a] Sources:
Calcium requirements. Report of a FAO/WHO Expert Committee. Geneva, World Health Organization, 1962 (WHO Technical Report Series, No. 230).
Requirements of vitamin A, iron, folate and vitamin B_{12}. Report of a Joint FAO/WHO Expert Consultation. Rome, Food and Agriculture Organization of the United Nations, 1988.
De Maeyer EM et al. *Preventing and controlling iron deficiency anaemia through primary health care.* Geneva, World Health Organization, 1989.
Trace elements in human nutrition and health. Geneva, World Health Organization, 1996.

[b] The second figure is for industrialized countries and represents intake levels to which the population is accustomed; the first is for developing countries, where body weight is lower and the population is adapted to lower levels of calcium intake that apparently do not give rise to disabilities.

[c] Iron requirements are calculated as follows:
very low: 4% (diets as in south Asia)
low: 7.5% (diets as in developing countries)
moderate: 15% (diets as in middle-income countries)
high: 22% (diets as in industrialized countries).

[d] The lower figure is for breast-fed infants, the higher for infants fed on breast-milk substitutes.

[e] The additional iron needed in the course of a pregnancy is about 1 gram. Some of this can come from the body's iron stores. However, in most cases these extra needs cannot be met from dietary sources, and iron supplementation is necessary. This is particularly important when bioavailability from the diet is poor.

ANNEX 2

Basic facts about food and nutrition

Types of nutrients

All foods are made up of five basic types of nutrients: carbohydrates, fats, proteins, vitamins, and minerals, plus variable amounts of water.

Carbohydrates

Carbohydrates are mostly starches and sugars of vegetable origin and a major component of, for example, cereals and tubers. In most poor countries, food energy is derived mainly from carbohydrate sources, especially cereals. In wealthy countries many people are advised to eat more cereals and potatoes.

Fats and oils

Fats and oils are also important sources of energy, having more than twice the energy content (weight for weight) of carbohydrates and proteins. In developing countries, however, fats account for a much smaller proportion of energy than carbohydrates. Fat consumption is often excessive in wealthy countries.

Proteins

Some proportion of protein is found in many human foods. Cereals, for example, contain about 8–12% protein, and beans contain twice as much. Some of the constituent amino acids of protein — the so-called essential amino acids — cannot be made by the body and must be obtained directly from food.

Proteins of animal origin, i.e. in milk, meat, eggs, cheese, fish, and poultry, contain all the essential amino acids in balanced amounts. Proteins of vegetable origin contain limited quantities of some of the essential amino acids. However, by combining different vegetable foods, e.g. cereals with pulses, or by adding some animal protein to vegetable sources, adequate protein levels (with all the essential amino acids in the right proportion) can be obtained. It is possible for people to obtain protein of adequate quality entirely from mixed vegetable sources, without eating any protein from animal sources.

Vitamins

Vitamins are needed for the adequate functioning of the body. There are two main groups:

- *Water-soluble vitamins.* This group comprises the B-complex vitamins — especially thiamine (B_1), riboflavin (B_2), and niacin — and vitamin C. Whole cereals, pulses and other vegetables, and animal foods are adequate sources of the B-complex vitamins, while vitamin C is found in raw fruits and vegetables. Water-soluble vitamins are relatively easily lost during cooking; losses are often as high as 60% and sometimes more (e.g. 90%), depending on the duration and temperature of cooking. Enough water, but no more, should be added for the cooking; any excess should be used in a sauce or soup.

- *Fat-soluble vitamins.* This group comprises vitamins A, D, E, and K, which are found in most animal products. The most important in emergencies are A and D. Significant amounts are stored in the body, especially in the liver, and vitamin A can also be produced in the body from the β-carotenes (provitamin A) that occur in most yellow and green leafy vegetables and orange-coloured fruits. Vitamin D is produced in the skin on exposure to sunlight, and is present in the liver of fish and animals and in some fortified foods from commercial sources (e.g. margarine).

Minerals

Iron is required for the formation of haemoglobin, and iron deficiency is a common cause of anaemia in many countries. Green leafy vegetables, red meats, and fish contain good amounts of iron, but its absorption from vegetable sources is very low; addition of even small amounts of animal foods and of vitamin C to the diet enhances iron absorption considerably. Tea or coffee drunk with meals inhibits absorption and should therefore be avoided.

Deficiency of sodium and potassium is likely to be seen only in individuals with severe diarrhoea. In such circumstances, sodium intake is increased by giving oral rehydration salt (ORS) solution. Potassium is present in large amounts in tubers, starchy fruits, and molasses. Several other minerals are essential to the diet, but are not usually critical in emergency situations.

Further information on trace elements and nutrition may be found in:

- *Trace elements in human nutrition and health.* Geneva, World Health Organization, 1996.

Water

For practical purposes, dietary water requirements may be considered to consist of the amount needed for replacement of the losses in urine, faeces, and perspiration. Young children are extremely vulnerable to dehydration (e.g. through diarrhoea, vomiting, sweating), which is associated with loss of salt and (if diarrhoea is prolonged) potassium.

The average minimum daily water requirements of healthy children in warm climates are approximately as follows:

- at 1 month: 400 ml (this amount can be wholly provided by breast milk)
- at 4 months: 600 ml (breast milk is still sufficient at this stage)
- at 12 months: 800 ml
- at 3 years: 1000 ml
- for older children (and adults) 1–1.5 litres

Nutritional priorities and vulnerable groups

When food is scarce, providing enough energy is the first priority of relief measures. If an individual does not consume enough energy, the body will begin to consume the protein that would normally be used for growth and repair. Eventually, muscle will be broken down.

Carbohydrates and fats provide the least expensive sources of energy, with fats being the densest source of energy:

- 1g of carbohydrates provides approximately 4 $kcal_{th}$
- 1g of fat provides approximately 9 $kcal_{th}$
- 1g of protein provides approximately 4 $kcal_{th}$.

Fats also improve the palatability of food and make it less viscous (softer and more runny). They also reduce the bulk required for a given energy intake (which are particularly important points for young children and in rehabilitation from severe malnutrition), and therefore reduce transport requirements. Ideally about 20% (minimum 15%, maximum 30%) of daily energy requirements should be supplied in the form of fats and oils.[1]

Particular consideration should be given to the needs of nutritionally vulnerable groups. Malnourished individuals, if they are to recover, require much higher levels of energy intake than healthy individuals of the same age. Pregnant women and women who are breast-feeding need extra calories and protein, and pregnant women need iron supplements.

Young children also need concentrated sources of energy and protein and require more frequent feeds or meals (three or four daily feedings) as they cannot eat or absorb large quantities at a time; they are especially vulnerable to infections and malnutrition. Their nutritional status thus requires close monitoring, especially in cultures in which children are served last and receive only whatever food remains after others have eaten.

When children are sick they should, if possible, be given more food rather than less. This includes breast milk, which is an important part of the diet of the infant and young child up to the age of 2 years or beyond, and should be the sole food for the first 4–6 months.

Foods and diets

If enough food is available to meet people's energy requirements, most local diets contain sufficient protein, and most other nutrients, to maintain health. The essential characteristics of a number of types of food are summarized in the following paragraphs, and Table A2.1 provides some details on the composition of common foods.

[1] See *Diet, nutrition, and the prevention of chronic diseases. Report of a WHO Study Group*, Geneva, World Health Organization, 1990 (WHO Technical Report Series, No. 797), and *Fats and oils in human nutrition. Report of a joint FAO/WHO expert consultation*, Rome, Food and Agriculture Organization of the United Nations, 1994 (Food and Nutrition Paper, No. 57).

Table A2.1 *Protein and energy content of some foods commonly consumed in tropical countries*[a]

Commodity (100-g edible portion, raw[b])	Energy content ($kcal_{th}$)	Protein content (g)	Waste[c] (g)
Cereals			
Rice			
Lightly milled (brown)	350	7	0
Overmilled (white or polished)	350	6	0
Parboiled	360	7	0
Wheat			
Bulgur wheat	380	11	0
Whole wheat:			
— soft	350	12	0
— hard	350	11	0
Flour	340	11.5	0
Wheat flour, 80% extraction rate	340	11	0
Maize, whole	350	9	0
Millet and sorghum	330	10	0
Vegetables and fruits			
Cassava leaves	90	4	20 or more
Fresh sweet potato leaves	50	4	20 or more
Fresh dark green leaves	50	2.5	20 or more
Carrots	40	1	10
Tomato	20	1	2
Fresh citrus fruits	40	0.5	25
Mango (ripe)	60	0.5	30–50
Papaya (ripe)	30	0.5	30
Dates:			
— raw	140	1	25
— dried	190	2	15
Fats and oils			
Butter	680	1.0	0
Ghee (butter oil)	850	—	0
Palm oil	900	—	0
Vegetable oil (others)	900	—	0
Pulses and oilseeds			
Lentils	340	20	0
Kidney beans	330	21	0
Peas	340	25	0
Chickpeas	350	20	0
Black and red beans	360	25	0
Nere (dried African locust bean)	400	32	70
Groundnuts:			
— shelled	550	23–26	2
— dried press-cake	380	36	
Soy beans:			
— dried seeds	400	33	0
— partially defatted flour	250	46	0
Cowpeas	340	23	0
Mung beans (green gram)	330	24	0
Starchy roots and fruits, tubers			
Cassava			
— fresh	150	0.5–1	15
— flour	340	1–2	0
Sweet potato (fresh, pale or orange)	110	1	15
Yams			
— tuber, fresh	110	2	15
— flour	320	4	0
— cocoyam	102	2	0

Table A2.1 (continued)

Commodity (100-g edible portion, raw[b])	Energy content ($kcal_{th}$)	Protein content (g)	Waste[c] (g)
Bananas			
— green	70	1	33
— ripe	120	1	33
— plantain bananas	130	1	33
Breadfruit (pulp, fresh)	90	1	25

[a] Adapted, with permission, from Platt BS. *Tables of representative values of foods commonly used in tropical countries.* London, Her Majesty's Stationery Office, 1975 (Medical Research Council Special Report Series, No. 302).

[b] The content of cooked food varies with the method of cooking and especially with the water content of the finished dish.

[c] "Waste" values are given as percentages of the food as purchased, but this proportion may vary widely.

Cereal grains

Cereal grains (rice, corn, millet, sorghum, oats, wheat, etc.) are staple foods and are the main source of energy in most cultures and of protein in many. They contain considerable amounts of protein (8–12%), B vitamins, and iron. However, most of the vitamins (especially thiamine) are lost in the milling process. The whiter the flour, the greater the loss of vitamins, and unless white flour is enriched or fortified with minerals and vitamins, it does not provide adequate micronutrients. About half of the remaining B vitamins are lost during cooking, and more if excess water is used and the surplus is discarded at the end of cooking. The "absorption" method of cooking avoids this loss. Yellow maize provides useful amounts of provitamin A.

Pulses and oilseeds

Dried pulses and oilseeds (mature beans, peas, soya, groundnuts, etc.) generally contain about 20% protein (soy beans, for example, are over 30% protein) and are rich in B vitamins and iron (although the iron is poorly absorbed). They are especially nutritious when they are eaten with cereals, since the proteins in the two groups complement each other. Pulses represent a concentrated form of energy. They are easier to digest when they are soaked overnight and the skins are removed. Careful storage is necessary to protect them from insects and rodents.

Tubers and roots

Tubers and roots (yams, taro, cassava, sweet potato, potato, etc.) provide mostly carbohydrates. Their protein content is low (0.5–2%) and they are bulky, so they are not suitable staples for feeding infants unless they are supplemented by other foods that are rich in protein and oil or fat. However, they do provide useful amounts of iron and B and C vitamins. Some orange varieties of sweet potato provide good quantities of provitamin A.

Vegetables and fruits

Vegetables and fruits contain a lot of water and few calories, but are often rich in provitamin A or carotenes, B and C vitamins, iron, and calcium. Dark-green leafy vegetables such as young cassava leaves and baobab leaves are especially good sources of these nutrients and also contain 2–4% protein.

Animal products

Animal products (meat, fish, eggs, and dairy products except butter) are excellent sources of complete, high-quality proteins. They are consumed in very small quantities in most developing countries, even under normal conditions, and may become even scarcer in emergencies. Even small amounts will significantly enhance the quality and palatability of a diet and the absorption of iron. Local taboos sometimes restrict their consumption by some groups such as young children and pregnant women.

Milks are rich in protein, sugar, fat, calcium, and vitamins, but poor in iron (although the iron in breast milk is well absorbed). Skim (non-fat) milk does not contain the fat-soluble vitamins A and D unless these are added during processing; this should be checked on the labelling.

Oils and fats

Oils and fats are concentrated sources of calories and also enhance the palatability of other foods. Fats derived from milk are rich in vitamins A and D; however, with the exception of red palm oil, which is extremely rich in provitamin A, vegetable oils do not contain vitamin A or D unless they have been appropriately fortified.

ANNEX 3

Nutritional anthropometry in emergencies

Introduction

This annex deals with the technical aspects of anthropometric assessments in emergencies. The parameters used for these assessments are discussed in Chapter 3.

The "gold standard" in anthropometric assessment of children is weight-for-length/height, with the usual practice being to measure the length of children under 2 years of age and the height of older children. It may be preferable, however, to use length measurements consistently. For most purposes, measurements are made on children from 6 months to 5 years (59 months) of age. Infants from birth to 5 months are included if moderate or severe maternal undernutrition or infections are suspected, and infant feeding practices (for infants from birth to 1 year) should in any case be assessed.

For measurements in small children, a weighing scale and a length-board are virtually essential items of equipment. It is possible to measure the height of children under 2 years old but this requires an extra assistant and is difficult to perform accurately. Length-boards are available through various agencies but may not be sufficiently robust for emergency situations. Locally made versions, using a design such as that shown in Fig. A3.2, are preferable. If age is not known exactly, the cut-off length corresponding to 2 years of age is 85 cm in non-stunted populations, but about 80 cm in chronically undernourished populations. For age 5 years, the corresponding cut-offs are 110 and 100 cm, respectively. Length-boards should therefore be at least 120 cm long. If older children are to be measured (for example, up to 10 years, with cut-offs of 137 and 130 cm), the length-boards should be 140 cm long; otherwise height may be determined using an adult height measure.

The internationally accepted WHO/NCHS reference values for weight-for-length/height up to 137 cm (10 years) are given in Table A3.1 for the two sexes separately and in Table A3.2 for the sexes combined.[1] Use of "combined" reference values will result in a slight underestimate of undernutrition in boys and an overestimate in girls and is therefore *not* generally recommended. However, under field conditions in emergencies, pressures of time and numbers of people may make it difficult to record sex reliably or to maintain separate records.

[1] WHO/NCHS growth reference data for height and weight of US children were originally collected by the National Center for Health Statistics (NCHS) and are recommended by WHO for international use.

***Table A3.1** WHO/NCHS normalized reference weight-for-length/height (49–137 cm) by sex*

Boys' weight (kg)					Length/ height (cm)	Girls' weight (kg)				
Median	−1 SD	−2 SD	−3 SD	−4 SD		Median	−1 SD	−2 SD	−3 SD	−4 SD
3.1	2.8	2.5	2.1	1.8	49	3.3	2.9	2.6	2.2	1.8
3.2	2.9	2.5	2.1	1.8	49.5	3.4	3.0	2.6	2.2	1.8
3.3	2.9	2.5	2.2	1.8	50	3.4	3.0	2.6	2.3	1.9
3.4	3.0	2.6	2.2	1.8	50.5	3.5	3.1	2.7	2.3	1.9
3.5	3.1	2.6	2.2	1.8	51	3.5	3.1	2.7	2.3	1.9
3.6	3.1	2.7	2.3	1.8	51.5	3.6	3.2	2.8	2.4	1.9
3.7	3.2	2.8	2.3	1.9	52	3.7	3.3	2.8	2.4	2.0
3.8	3.3	2.8	2.4	1.9	52.5	3.8	3.4	2.9	2.5	2.0
3.9	3.4	2.9	2.4	1.9	53	3.9	3.4	3.0	2.5	2.1
4.0	3.5	3.0	2.5	2.0	53.5	4.0	3.5	3.1	2.6	2.1
4.1	3.6	3.1	2.6	2.0	54	4.1	3.6	3.1	2.7	2.2
4.2	3.7	3.2	2.6	2.1	54.5	4.2	3.7	3.2	2.7	2.2
4.3	3.8	3.3	2.7	2.2	55	4.3	3.8	3.3	2.8	2.3
4.5	3.9	3.3	2.8	2.2	55.5	4.4	3.9	3.4	2.9	2.4
4.6	4.0	3.5	2.9	2.3	56	4.5	4.0	3.5	3.0	2.4
4.7	4.1	3.6	3.0	2.4	56.5	4.6	4.1	3.6	3.0	2.5
4.8	4.3	3.7	3.1	2.5	57	4.8	4.2	3.7	3.1	2.6
5.0	4.4	3.8	3.2	2.6	57.5	4.9	4.3	3.8	3.2	2.7
5.1	4.5	3.9	3.3	2.7	58	5.0	4.4	3.9	3.3	2.7
5.2	4.6	4.0	3.4	2.8	58.5	5.1	4.6	4.0	3.4	2.8
5.4	4.8	4.1	3.5	2.9	59	5.3	4.7	4.1	3.5	2.9
5.5	4.9	4.2	3.6	3.0	59.5	5.4	4.8	4.2	3.6	3.0
5.7	5.0	4.4	3.7	3.1	60	5.5	4.9	4.3	3.7	3.1
5.8	5.1	4.5	3.8	3.2	60.5	5.7	5.1	4.4	3.8	3.2
5.9	5.3	4.6	4.0	3.3	61	5.8	5.2	4.6	3.9	3.3
6.1	5.4	4.8	4.1	3.4	61.5	6.0	5.3	4.7	4.0	3.4
6.2	5.6	4.9	4.2	3.5	62	6.1	5.4	4.8	4.1	3.5
6.4	5.7	5.0	4.3	3.7	62.5	6.2	5.6	4.9	4.2	3.6
6.5	5.8	5.2	4.5	3.8	63	6.4	5.7	5.0	4.4	3.7
6.7	6.0	5.3	4.6	3.9	63.5	6.5	5.8	5.2	4.5	3.8
6.8	6.1	5.4	4.7	4.0	64	6.7	6.0	5.3	4.6	3.9
7.0	6.3	5.6	4.9	4.2	64.5	6.8	6.1	5.4	4.7	4.0
7.1	6.4	5.7	5.0	4.3	65	7.0	6.3	5.5	4.8	4.1
7.3	6.5	5.8	5.1	4.4	65.5	7.1	6.4	5.7	4.9	4.2
7.4	6.7	6.0	5.3	4.5	66	7.3	6.5	5.8	5.1	4.3
7.6	6.8	6.1	5.4	4.7	66.5	7.4	6.7	5.9	5.2	4.4
7.7	7.0	6.2	5.5	4.8	67	7.5	6.8	6.0	5.3	4.5
7.8	7.1	6.4	5.7	4.9	67.5	7.7	6.9	6.2	5.4	4.7
8.0	7.3	6.5	5.8	5.1	68	7.8	7.1	6.3	5.5	4.8
8.1	7.4	6.6	5.9	5.2	68.5	8.0	7.2	6.4	5.6	4.9
8.3	7.5	6.8	6.0	5.3	69	8.1	7.3	6.5	5.8	5.0
8.4	7.7	6.9	6.2	5.4	69.5	8.2	7.5	6.7	5.9	5.1
8.5	7.8	7.0	6.3	5.5	70	8.4	7.6	6.8	6.0	5.2
8.7	7.9	7.2	6.4	5.7	70.5	8.5	7.7	6.9	6.1	5.3
8.8	8.1	7.3	6.5	5.8	71	8.6	7.8	7.0	6.2	5.4
8.9	8.2	7.4	6.7	5.9	71.5	8.8	8.0	7.1	6.3	5.5
9.1	8.3	7.5	6.8	6.0	72	8.9	8.1	7.2	6.4	5.6
9.2	8.4	7.7	6.9	6.1	72.5	9.0	8.2	7.4	6.5	5.7
9.3	8.6	7.8	7.0	6.2	73	9.1	8.3	7.5	6.6	5.8
9.5	8.7	7.9	7.1	6.3	73.5	9.3	8.4	7.6	6.7	5.9
9.6	8.8	8.0	7.2	6.4	74	9.4	8.5	7.7	6.8	6.0
9.7	8.9	8.1	7.3	6.5	74.5	9.5	8.6	7.8	6.9	6.1
9.8	9.0	8.2	7.4	6.6	75	9.6	8.7	7.9	7.0	6.2
9.9	9.1	8.3	7.5	6.7	75.5	9.7	8.8	8.0	7.1	6.3
10.0	9.2	8.4	7.6	6.8	76	9.8	8.9	8.1	7.2	6.4
10.2	9.3	8.5	7.7	6.9	76.5	9.9	9.0	8.2	7.3	6.5
10.3	9.4	8.6	7.8	7.0	77	10.0	9.1	8.3	7.4	6.6

Table A3.1 *(continued)*

Boys' weight (kg)					Length/ height (cm)	Girls' weight (kg)				
Median	−1 SD	−2 SD	−3 SD	−4 SD		Median	−1 SD	−2 SD	−3 SD	−4 SD
10.4	9.5	8.7	7.9	7.1	77.5	10.1	9.2	8.4	7.5	6.6
10.5	9.7	8.8	8.0	7.1	78	10.2	9.3	8.5	7.6	6.7
10.6	9.8	8.9	8.1	7.2	78.5	10.3	9.4	8.6	7.7	6.8
10.7	9.9	9.0	8.2	7.3	79	10.4	9.5	8.7	7.8	6.9
10.8	10.0	9.1	8.2	7.4	79.5	10.5	9.6	8.7	7.9	7.0
10.9	10.1	9.2	8.3	7.5	80	10.6	9.7	8.8	8.0	7.1
11.0	10.1	9.3	8.4	7.6	80.5	10.7	9.8	8.9	8.0	7.2
11.1	10.2	9.4	8.5	7.6	81	10.8	9.9	9.0	8.1	7.2
11.2	10.3	9.5	8.6	7.7	81.5	10.9	10.0	9.1	8.2	7.3
11.3	10.4	9.6	8.7	7.8	82	11.0	10.1	9.2	8.3	7.4
11.4	10.5	9.6	8.8	7.9	82.5	11.1	10.2	9.3	8.4	7.5
11.5	10.6	9.7	8.8	7.9	83	11.2	10.3	9.4	8.5	7.6
11.6	10.7	9.8	8.9	8.0	83.5	11.3	10.4	9.5	8.6	7.7
11.7	10.8	9.9	9.0	8.1	84	11.4	10.5	9.6	8.7	7.7
11.8	10.9	10.0	9.1	8.2	84.5	11.5	10.6	9.6	8.7	7.8
12.1	11.0	9.9	8.9	7.8	85	11.8	10.8	9.7	8.6	7.6
12.2	11.1	10.0	8.9	7.9	85.5	11.9	10.9	9.8	8.7	7.6
12.3	11.2	10.1	9.0	7.9	86	12.0	11.0	9.9	8.8	7.7
12.5	11.3	10.2	9.1	8.0	86.5	12.2	11.1	10.0	8.9	7.8
12.6	11.5	10.3	9.2	8.1	87	12.3	11.2	10.1	9.0	7.9
12.7	11.6	10.4	9.3	8.2	87.5	12.4	11.3	10.2	9.1	8.0
12.8	11.7	10.5	9.4	8.3	88	12.5	11.4	10.3	9.2	8.1
12.9	11.8	10.6	9.5	8.4	88.5	12.6	11.5	10.4	9.3	8.1
13.0	11.9	10.7	9.6	8.4	89	12.7	11.6	10.5	9.3	8.2
13.1	12.0	10.8	9.7	8.5	89.5	12.8	11.7	10.6	9.4	8.3
13.3	12.1	10.9	9.8	8.6	90	12.9	11.8	10.7	9.5	8.4
13.4	12.2	11.0	9.9	8.7	90.5	13.0	11.9	10.7	9.6	8.5
13.5	12.3	11.1	9.9	8.8	91	13.2	12.0	10.8	9.7	8.5
13.6	12.4	11.2	10.0	8.8	91.5	13.3	12.1	10.9	9.8	8.6
13.7	12.5	11.3	10.1	8.9	92	13.4	12.2	11.0	9.9	8.7
13.9	12.6	11.4	10.2	9.0	92.5	13.5	12.3	11.1	9.9	8.8
14.0	12.8	11.5	10.3	9.1	93	13.6	12.4	11.2	10.0	8.8
14.1	12.9	11.6	10.4	9.2	93.5	13.7	12.5	11.3	10.1	8.9
14.2	13.0	11.7	10.5	9.2	94	13.9	12.6	11.4	10.2	9.0
14.3	13.1	11.8	10.6	9.3	94.5	14.0	12.8	11.5	10.3	9.1
14.5	13.2	11.9	10.7	9.4	95	14.1	12.9	11.6	10.4	9.1
14.6	13.3	12.0	10.8	9.5	95.5	14.2	13.0	11.7	10.5	9.2
14.7	13.4	12.1	10.9	9.6	96	14.3	13.1	11.8	10.6	9.3
14.8	13.5	12.2	11.0	9.7	96.5	14.5	13.2	11.9	10.7	9.4
15.0	13.7	12.4	11.0	9.7	97	14.6	13.3	12.0	10.7	9.5
15.1	13.8	12.5	11.1	9.8	97.5	14.7	13.4	12.1	10.8	9.5
15.2	13.9	12.6	11.2	9.9	98	14.9	13.5	12.2	10.9	9.6
15.4	14.0	12.7	11.3	10.0	98.5	15.0	13.7	12.3	11.0	9.7
15.5	14.1	12.8	11.4	10.1	99	15.1	13.8	12.4	11.1	9.8
15.6	14.3	12.9	11.5	10.2	99.5	15.2	13.9	12.5	11.2	9.9
15.7	14.4	13.0	11.6	10.3	100	15.4	14.0	12.7	11.3	9.9
15.9	14.5	13.1	11.7	10.3	100.5	15.5	14.1	12.8	11.4	10.0
16.0	14.6	13.2	11.8	10.4	101	15.6	14.3	12.9	11.5	10.1
16.2	14.7	13.3	11.9	10.5	101.5	15.8	14.4	13.0	11.6	10.2
16.3	14.9	13.4	12.0	10.6	102	15.9	14.5	13.1	11.7	10.3
16.4	15.0	13.6	12.1	10.7	102.5	16.0	14.6	13.2	11.8	10.4
16.6	15.1	13.7	12.2	10.8	103	16.2	14.7	13.3	11.9	10.5
16.7	15.3	13.8	12.3	10.9	103.5	16.3	14.9	13.4	12.0	10.5
16.9	15.4	13.9	12.4	11.0	104	16.5	15.0	13.5	12.1	10.6
17.0	15.5	14.0	12.6	11.1	104.5	16.6	15.1	13.7	12.2	10.7
17.1	15.6	14.2	12.7	11.2	105	16.7	15.3	13.8	12.3	10.8
17.3	15.8	14.3	12.8	11.3	105.5	16.9	15.4	13.9	12.4	10.9

Table A3.1 *(continued)*

Boys' weight (kg)					Length/ height (cm)	Girls' weight (kg)				
Median	−1 SD	−2 SD	−3 SD	−4 SD		Median	−1 SD	−2 SD	−3 SD	−4 SD
17.4	15.9	14.4	12.9	11.4	106	17.0	15.5	14.0	12.5	11.0
17.6	16.1	14.5	13.0	11.5	106.5	17.2	15.7	14.1	12.6	11.1
17.7	16.2	14.7	13.1	11.6	107	17.3	15.8	14.3	12.7	11.2
17.9	16.3	14.8	13.2	11.7	107.5	17.5	15.9	14.4	12.8	11.3
18.0	16.5	14.9	13.4	11.8	108	17.6	16.1	14.5	13.0	11.4
18.2	16.6	15.0	13.5	11.9	108.5	17.8	16.2	14.6	13.1	11.5
18.3	16.8	15.2	13.6	12.0	109	17.9	16.4	14.8	13.2	11.6
18.5	16.9	15.3	13.7	12.1	109.5	18.1	16.5	14.9	13.3	11.7
18.7	17.1	15.4	13.8	12.2	110	18.2	16.6	15.0	13.4	11.9
18.8	17.2	15.6	14.0	12.3	110.5	18.4	16.8	15.2	13.6	12.0
19.0	17.4	15.7	14.1	12.5	111	18.6	16.9	15.3	13.7	12.1
19.1	17.5	15.9	14.2	12.6	111.5	18.7	17.1	15.5	13.8	12.2
19.3	17.7	16.0	14.4	12.7	112	18.9	17.2	15.6	14.0	12.3
19.5	17.8	16.1	14.5	12.8	112.5	19.0	17.4	15.7	14.1	12.4
19.6	18.0	16.3	14.6	12.9	113	19.2	17.5	15.9	14.2	12.6
19.8	18.1	16.4	14.8	13.1	113.5	19.4	17.7	16.0	14.4	12.7
20.0	18.3	16.6	14.9	13.2	114	19.5	17.9	16.2	14.5	12.8
20.2	18.5	16.7	15.0	13.3	114.5	19.7	18.0	16.3	14.6	12.9
20.3	18.6	16.9	15.2	13.5	115	19.9	18.2	16.5	14.8	13.0
20.5	18.8	17.1	15.3	13.6	115.5	20.1	18.4	16.6	14.9	13.2
20.7	18.9	17.2	15.5	13.7	116	20.3	18.5	16.8	15.0	13.3
20.9	19.1	17.4	15.6	13.9	116.5	20.4	18.7	16.9	15.2	13.4
21.1	19.3	17.5	15.8	14.0	117	20.6	18.9	17.1	15.3	13.6
21.2	19.5	17.7	15.9	14.2	117.5	20.8	19.0	17.3	15.5	13.7
21.4	19.6	17.9	16.1	14.3	118	21.0	19.2	17.4	15.6	13.8
21.6	19.8	18.0	16.2	14.4	118.5	21.2	19.4	17.6	15.8	13.9
21.8	20.0	18.2	16.4	14.6	119	21.4	19.6	17.7	15.9	14.1
22.0	20.2	18.4	16.6	14.7	119.5	21.6	19.8	17.9	16.1	14.2
22.2	20.4	18.5	16.7	14.9	120	21.8	20.0	18.1	16.2	14.3
22.4	20.6	18.7	16.9	15.0	120.5	22.0	20.1	18.3	16.4	14.5
22.6	20.7	18.9	17.0	15.2	121	22.2	20.3	18.4	16.5	14.6
22.8	20.9	19.1	17.2	15.3	121.5	22.5	20.5	18.6	16.7	14.7
23.0	21.1	19.2	17.4	15.5	122	22.7	20.7	18.8	16.8	14.9
23.2	21.3	19.4	17.5	15.6	122.5	22.9	20.9	19.0	17.0	15.0
23.4	21.5	19.6	17.7	15.8	123	23.1	21.1	19.1	17.1	15.1
23.6	21.7	19.8	17.9	16.0	123.5	23.4	21.3	19.3	17.3	15.3
23.9	21.9	20.0	18.0	16.1	124	23.6	21.6	19.5	17.4	15.4
24.1	22.1	20.2	18.2	16.3	124.5	23.9	21.8	19.7	17.6	15.5
24.3	22.3	20.4	18.4	16.4	125	24.1	22.0	19.9	17.8	15.6
24.5	22.5	20.5	18.6	16.6	125.5	24.3	22.2	20.1	17.9	15.8
24.8	22.8	20.7	18.7	16.7	126	24.6	22.4	20.2	18.1	15.9
25.0	23.0	20.9	18.9	16.9	126.5	24.9	22.7	20.4	18.2	16.0
25.2	23.2	21.1	19.1	17.0	127	25.1	22.9	20.6	18.4	16.2
25.5	23.4	21.3	19.2	17.2	127.5	25.4	23.1	20.8	18.6	16.3
25.7	23.6	21.5	19.4	17.3	128	25.7	23.3	21.0	18.7	16.4
26.0	23.8	21.7	19.6	17.5	128.5	25.9	23.6	21.2	18.9	16.5
26.2	24.1	21.9	19.8	17.6	129	26.2	23.8	21.4	19.0	16.7
26.5	24.3	22.1	19.9	17.7	129.5	26.5	24.1	21.6	19.2	16.8
26.8	24.5	22.3	20.1	17.9	130	26.8	24.3	21.8	19.4	16.9
27.0	24.8	22.5	20.3	18.0	130.5	27.1	24.6	22.1	19.5	17.0
27.3	25.0	22.7	20.4	18.2	131	27.4	24.8	22.3	19.7	17.1
27.6	25.2	22.9	20.6	18.3	131.5	27.7	25.1	22.5	19.9	17.2
27.8	25.5	23.1	20.8	18.4	132	28.0	25.4	22.7	20.0	17.4
28.1	25.7	23.3	21.0	18.6	132.5	28.4	25.6	22.9	20.2	17.5
28.4	26.0	23.6	21.1	18.7	133	28.7	25.9	23.1	20.4	17.6
28.7	26.2	23.8	21.3	18.8	133.5	29.0	26.2	23.4	20.5	17.7
29.0	26.5	24.0	21.5	18.9	134	29.4	26.5	23.6	20.7	17.8

Table A3.1 *(continued)*

Boys' weight (kg)					Length/ height (cm)	Girls' weight (kg)				
Median	**−1 SD**	**−2 SD**	**−3 SD**	**−4 SD**		**Median**	**−1 SD**	**−2 SD**	**−3 SD**	**−4 SD**
29.3	26.7	24.2	21.6	19.1	134.5	29.7	26.8	23.8	20.8	17.9
29.6	27.0	24.4	21.8	19.2	135	30.1	27.0	24.0	21.0	18.0
29.9	27.3	24.6	22.0	19.3	135.5	30.4	27.3	24.3	21.2	18.1
30.2	27.5	24.8	22.1	19.4	136	30.8	27.6	24.5	21.3	18.2
30.6	27.8	25.0	22.3	19.5	136.5	31.1	27.9	24.7	21.5	18.3
30.9	28.1	25.3	22.4	19.6	137	31.5	28.2	25.0	21.7	18.4

Notes:

1. Length is generally measured in children below 85 cm and height in children 85 cm and above. Recumbent length is on average 0.5 cm greater than standing height; although the difference is of no importance to the individual child, a correction may be made by deducting 0.5 cm from all lengths above 84.9 cm if standing height cannot be measured.
2. SD = standard deviation score (or Z-score). The relationship between the percentage-of-median value and the SD-score or Z-score varies with age and height, particularly in the first year of life, and beyond 5 years. Between 1 and 5 years median −1 SD and median −2 SD correspond to approximately 90% and 80% of median (weight-for-length/height, and weight-for-age), respectively. Beyond 5 years of age or 110 cm (or 100 cm in stunted children) this equivalence is not maintained; median −2 SD is much below 80% of median. Hence the use of "percentage-of-median" is not recommended, particularly in children of school age. Somewhere beyond 10 years or 137 cm, the adolescent growth spurt begins and the time of its onset is variable. The correct interpretation of weight-for-height data beyond this point is therefore difficult.

Table A3.2 *WHO/NCHS normalized reference weight-for-length/height (58–137 cm) for the sexes combined*

Length/ height (cm)	Weight (kg)		Length/ height (cm)	Weight (kg)	
	Median −2 SD	**Median −3 SD**		**Median −2 SD**	**Median −3 SD**
58	3.9	3.3	71.5	7.3	6.5
58.5	4.0	3.4	72	7.4	6.6
59	4.1	3.5	72.5	7.6	6.7
59.5	4.2	3.6	73	7.7	6.8
60	4.4	3.7	73.5	7.8	6.9
60.5	4.5	3.8	74	7.9	7.0
61	4.6	4.0	74.5	8.0	7.1
61.5	4.8	4.1	75	8.1	7.2
62	4.9	4.2	75.5	8.2	7.3
62.5	5.0	4.3	76	8.3	7.4
63	5.1	4.4	76.5	8.4	7.5
63.5	5.3	4.6	77	8.5	7.6
64	5.4	4.7	77.5	8.6	7.7
64.5	5.5	4.8	78	8.7	7.8
65	5.6	4.9	78.5	8.8	7.9
65.5	5.8	5.0	79	8.9	8.0
66	5.9	5.2	79.5	8.9	8.1
66.5	6.0	5.3	80	9.0	8.2
67	6.1	5.4	80.5	9.1	8.2
67.5	6.3	5.6	81	9.2	8.3
68	6.4	5.7	81.5	9.3	8.4
68.5	6.5	5.8	82	9.4	8.5
69	6.7	5.9	82.5	9.5	8.6
69.5	6.8	6.1	83	9.6	8.7
70	6.9	6.2	83.5	9.7	8.8
70.5	7.0	6.3	84	9.8	8.9
71	7.2	6.4	84.5	9.8	8.9

Table A3.2 (continued)

Length/ height (cm)	Weight (kg)		Length/ height (cm)	Weight (kg)	
	Median −2 SD	Median −3 SD		Median −2 SD	Median −3 SD
85	9.8	8.8	111.5	15.7	14.0
85.5	9.9	8.8	112	15.8	14.2
86	10.0	8.9	112.5	15.9	14.3
86.5	10.1	9.0	113	16.1	14.4
87	10.2	9.1	113.5	16.2	14.6
87.5	10.3	9.2	114	16.3	14.7
88	10.4	9.3	114.5	16.4	14.8
88.5	10.5	9.4	115	16.7	15.0
89	10.6	9.5	115.5	16.9	15.1
89.5	10.7	9.6	116	17.0	15.3
90	10.8	9.7	116.5	17.2	15.4
90.5	10.9	9.8	117	17.3	15.6
91	11.0	9.8	117.5	17.5	15.7
91.5	11.1	9.9	118	17.7	15.9
92	11.2	10.0	118.5	17.8	16.0
92.5	11.3	10.1	119	18.0	16.2
93	11.4	10.2	119.5	18.2	16.4
93.5	11.5	10.3	120	18.3	16.5
94	11.6	10.4	120.5	18.5	16.7
94.5	11.7	10.5	121	18.7	16.8
95	11.8	10.6	121.5	18.9	17.0
95.5	11.9	10.7	122	19.0	17.1
96	12.0	10.8	122.5	19.2	17.3
96.5	12.1	10.9	123	19.4	17.4
97	12.2	10.9	123.5	19.6	17.6
97.5	12.3	11.0	124	19.8	17.7
98	12.4	11.1	124.5	20.0	17.9
98.5	12.5	11.2	125	20.2	18.1
99	12.6	11.3	125.5	20.3	18.3
99.5	12.7	11.4	126	20.5	18.4
100	12.9	11.5	126.5	20.7	18.6
100.5	13.0	11.6	127	20.9	18.8
101	13.1	11.7	127.5	21.1	19.0
101.5	13.2	11.8	128	21.3	19.1
102	13.3	11.9	128.5	21.5	19.3
102.5	13.4	12.0	129	21.7	19.4
103	13.5	12.1	129.5	21.9	19.6
103.5	13.6	12.2	130	22.1	19.8
104	13.7	12.3	130.5	22.3	19.9
104.5	13.9	12.4	131	22.5	20.1
105	14.0	12.5	131.5	22.7	20.3
105.5	14.1	12.6	132	22.9	20.4
106	14.2	12.7	132.5	23.1	20.6
106.5	14.3	12.8	133	23.4	20.8
107	14.5	12.9	133.5	23.6	20.9
107.5	14.6	13.0	134	23.7	21.1
108	14.7	13.2	134.5	24.0	21.2
108.5	14.8	13.2	135	24.2	21.4
109	15.0	13.4	135.5	24.5	21.6
109.5	15.1	13.5	136	24.7	21.7
110	15.2	13.6	136.5	24.9	21.9
110.5	15.4	13.8	137	25.2	22.1
111	15.5	13.9			

Table A3.3 gives the values for one standard deviation of the WHO/NCHS reference median weight-for-length/height for each 0.5 cm of length/height up to 137 cm. The best index of a child's anthropometric status (in an emergency situation) is weight-for-length/height expressed in terms of Z-scores, where Z-score is defined as the deviation of the value for an individual from the median value of the reference population, divided by the standard deviation for the reference population:

$$\text{Z-score} = \frac{(\text{individual's value}) - (\text{median reference value})}{\text{standard deviation of reference population}}$$

Example

A girl of length 65 cm has a weight of 6.0 kg. Table A3.1 shows that reference median weight for this length is 7.0 kg and that the girl's weight lies between median−1 SD (6.3 kg) and median−2 SD (5.5 kg). Table A3.3 shows that the standard deviation of the reference median weight for length 65 cm is 0.715. Z-score can therefore be calculated as follows:

$$(6.0 - 7.0)/0.715 = -1.0/0.715 = -1.40$$

Table A3.3 *Values for one standard deviation of WHO/NCHS reference median weight-for-length/height*

Length/ height (cm)	One SD of median weight (kg)		Length/ height (cm)	One SD of median weight (kg)	
	Male	Female		Male	Female
49	0.341	0.365	64.5	0.700	0.705
49.5	0.362	0.375	65	0.705	0.715
50	0.382	0.386	65.5	0.710	0.724
50.5	0.401	0.397	66	0.715	0.733
51	0.420	0.409	66.5	0.720	0.742
51.5	0.438	0.420	67	0.724	0.751
52	0.455	0.431	67.5	0.729	0.759
52.5	0.471	0.442	68	0.733	0.767
53	0.487	0.454	68.5	0.738	0.775
53.5	0.502	0.465	69	0.742	0.783
54	0.516	0.477	69.5	0.747	0.791
54.5	0.529	0.488	70	0.751	0.798
55	0.542	0.499	70.5	0.756	0.804
55.5	0.555	0.511	71	0.760	0.811
56	0.567	0.522	71.5	0.765	0.817
56.5	0.578	0.534	72	0.770	0.823
57	0.589	0.545	72.5	0.774	0.829
57.5	0.599	0.556	73	0.779	0.834
58	0.608	0.568	73.5	0.785	0.839
58.5	0.618	0.579	74	0.790	0.844
59	0.627	0.590	74.5	0.795	0.848
59.5	0.635	0.601	75	0.801	0.852
60	0.643	0.612	75.5	0.806	0.856
60.5	0.651	0.623	76	0.812	0.860
61	0.658	0.634	76.5	0.818	0.863
61.5	0.665	0.644	77	0.823	0.867
62	0.671	0.655	77.5	0.829	0.870
62.5	0.678	0.665	78	0.835	0.873
63	0.684	0.676	78.5	0.841	0.876
63.5	0.689	0.686	79	0.847	0.879
64	0.695	0.696	79.5	0.853	0.881

Table A3.3 *(continued)*

Length/ height (cm)	One SD of median weight (kg)		Length/ height (cm)	One SD of median weight (kg)	
	Male	Female		Male	Female
80	0.859	0.884	109	1.584	1.574
80.5	0.865	0.887	109.5	1.595	1.585
81	0.871	0.889	110	1.607	1.596
81.5	0.877	0.892	110.5	1.618	1.607
82	0.884	0.894	111	1.629	1.618
82.5	0.890	0.897	111.5	1.641	1.629
83	0.896	0.900	112	1.652	1.640
83.5	0.902	0.902	112.5	1.663	1.652
84	0.908	0.905	113	1.674	1.663
84.5	0.914	0.908	113.5	1.685	1.675
85	1.087	1.069	114	1.696	1.687
85.5	1.094	1.074	114.5	1.707	1.700
86	1.101	1.080	115	1.717	1.713
86.5	1.108	1.086	115.5	1.728	1.726
87	1.116	1.092	116	1.738	1.740
87.5	1.124	1.099	116.5	1.749	1.754
88	1.132	1.106	117	1.759	1.769
88.5	1.140	1.114	117.5	1.770	1.784
89	1.148	1.122	118	1.780	1.800
89.5	1.157	1.130	118.5	1.791	1.817
90	1.166	1.138	119	1.803	1.834
90.5	1.175	1.147	119.5	1.814	1.852
91	1.184	1.156	120	1.826	1.871
91.5	1.194	1.166	120.5	1.838	1.891
92	1.203	1.176	121	1.851	1.911
92.5	1.213	1.186	121.5	1.864	1.933
93	1.223	1.196	122	1.878	1.955
93.5	1.233	1.206	122.5	1.892	1.979
94	1.243	1.217	123	1.907	2.003
94.5	1.253	1.228	123.5	1.923	2.029
95	1.264	1.239	124	1.940	2.056
95.5	1.274	1.250	124.5	1.957	2.083
96	1.285	1.262	125	1.975	2.113
96.5	1.296	1.273	125.5	1.994	2.143
97	1.306	1.285	126	2.015	2.175
97.5	1.317	1.297	126.5	2.036	2.207
98	1.329	1.309	127	2.058	2.242
98.5	1.340	1.321	127.5	2.082	2.278
99	1.351	1.333	128	2.106	2.315
99.5	1.362	1.345	128.5	2.132	2.353
100	1.374	1.358	129	2.159	2.394
100.5	1.385	1.370	129.5	2.188	2.435
101	1.397	1.382	130	2.218	2.479
101.5	1.408	1.395	130.5	2.249	2.524
102	1.420	1.407	131	2.282	2.571
102.5	1.431	1.419	131.5	2.317	2.619
103	1.443	1.432	132	2.353	2.670
103.5	1.455	1.444	132.5	2.391	2.722
104	1.467	1.456	133	2.430	2.776
104.5	1.478	1.469	133.5	2.472	2.832
105	1.490	1.481	134	2.515	2.890
105.5	1.502	1.493	134.5	2.560	2.950
106	1.513	1.505	135	2.607	3.012
106.5	1.525	1.517	135.5	2.656	3.076
107	1.537	1.528	136	2.707	3.142
107.5	1.549	1.540	136.5	2.760	3.210
108	1.560	1.551	137	2.815	3.281
108.5	1.572	1.563			

Using the Z-score for groups or communities

Calculating the mean Z-score for a community, on the basis of the individual Z-scores of all individuals studied, provides a measure of the severity of protein–energy malnutrition in the community. For this mean Z-score, a standard deviation and standard error of the mean (SEM) can be calculated (using a computer or the usual statistical formulae). The confidence interval, beyond which any values would be significantly different from the mean Z-score, is calculated as ($2 \times$ SEM). This provides a simple method for determining whether the Z-scores of two (or more) communities are significantly different from one another, or whether the Z-score of a particular community has changed significantly over a specifed period of time.

Example

A community has a mean Z-score of -0.5. Table 20 (page 40) shows that this community will be classed as being in "poor" condition. The calculated SEM was, say, 0.1. Only if an earlier Z-score was outside the range -0.5 ± 0.2, i.e. not between -0.3 and -0.7, has there been any *significant* change. Moreover, the condition of this community is not significantly different from that of any other community with a mean Z-score in the range -0.3 to -0.7 (and a similar value of SEM).

Use of mean Z-scores and SEMs provides more sensitive statistical comparisons of communities than percentages of populations below given cut-off values, and mean Z-score is ultimately a better indicator of the nutritional status of a particular community than the percentage of individuals below a conventional cut-off.

If any of the necessary equipment for determining weight and length/height is unavailable, as it may be in an emergency situation, MUAC measurements may be used instead — either MUAC-for-age or MUAC-for-length/height. Otherwise, use of MUAC for nutritional assessment offers no advantages. At one time, a single cut-off point (or two points at most) was used to cover the whole age interval from 6 months to 5 years. However, because there is normally a perceptible increase in MUAC (of 2–3 cm) over this period, many false conclusions were being drawn, with overestimates of undernutrition in younger children and underestimates in older children. (Other shortcomings of MUAC assessments are mentioned in Chapter 3, page 39). New WHO/NCHS reference values for MUAC-for-age have been developed;[1] these are presented in Table A3.4, together with cut-offs at -2 SD and -3 SD. Table A3.5 provides reference values for MUAC-for-length/height, also with cut-offs at -2 SD and -3 SD.[2]

Since the standards for boys and girls differ substantially up to about 1½ years of age, the sex of each child should normally be recorded and the data analysed separately. However, there may be circumstances in which this is not possible, and Tables A3.4 and A3.5 therefore include reference values for boys, for girls, and for the sexes combined.

---

[1] de Onis M, Yip R, Mei Z. The development of MUAC-for-age reference data: recommended by a WHO Expert Committee. *Bulletin of the World Health Organization*, 1997, 75(1):11–18.

[2] Mei Z et al. The development of a MUAC-for-height reference, including a comparison to other status screening indicators. *Bulletin of the World Health Organization*, 1997, 75(4):333–341.

Table A3.4 *WHO/NCHS normalized reference values for MUAC-for-age (6–59 months)*

Age (months)	Boys			Combined sexes			Girls		
	Median	−2SD	−3SD	Median	−2SD	−3SD	Median	−2SD	−3SD
6	14.9	12.6	11.5	14.3	12.0	10.9	13.9	11.5	10.4
7	15.1	12.7	11.6	14.6	12.2	11.0	14.1	11.8	10.6
8	15.2	12.8	11.7	14.8	12.4	11.2	14.4	12.0	10.8
9	15.4	12.9	11.7	14.9	12.5	11.3	14.6	12.2	11.0
10	15.5	13.0	11.8	15.1	12.7	11.5	14.8	12.3	11.1
11	15.6	13.1	11.9	15.2	12.8	11.6	15.0	12.5	11.3
12	15.7	13.2	11.9	15.4	12.9	11.7	15.1	12.6	11.4
13	15.7	13.2	12.0	15.5	13.0	11.7	15.2	12.7	11.5
14	15.8	13.3	12.0	15.6	13.1	11.8	15.4	12.8	11.6
15	15.9	13.3	12.1	15.7	13.1	11.9	15.5	12.9	11.7
16	15.9	13.4	12.1	15.8	13.2	11.9	15.6	13.0	11.7
17	16.0	13.4	12.1	15.8	13.2	12.0	15.7	13.1	11.8
18	16.0	13.4	12.1	15.9	13.3	12.0	15.7	13.1	11.8
19	16.1	13.5	12.2	15.9	13.3	12.0	15.8	13.2	11.9
20	16.1	13.5	12.2	16.0	13.4	12.1	15.8	13.2	11.9
21	16.1	13.5	12.2	16.0	13.4	12.1	15.9	13.3	11.9
22	16.2	13.5	12.2	16.1	13.4	12.1	15.9	13.3	12.0
23	16.2	13.5	12.2	16.1	13.4	12.1	16.0	13.3	12.0
24	16.2	13.6	12.2	16.1	13.5	12.1	16.0	13.4	12.0
25	16.3	13.6	12.2	16.2	13.5	12.2	16.1	13.4	12.0
26	16.3	13.6	12.3	16.2	13.5	12.2	16.1	13.4	12.1
27	16.3	13.6	12.3	16.2	13.5	12.2	16.1	13.4	12.1
28	16.3	13.6	12.3	16.3	13.5	12.2	16.1	13.4	12.1
29	16.4	13.7	12.3	16.3	13.6	12.2	16.2	13.5	12.1
30	16.4	13.7	12.3	16.3	13.6	12.2	16.2	13.5	12.1
31	16.4	13.7	12.3	16.3	13.6	12.2	16.2	13.5	12.1
32	16.5	13.7	12.3	16.4	13.6	12.2	16.3	13.5	12.1
33	16.5	13.7	12.4	16.4	13.6	12.3	16.3	13.5	12.2
34	16.5	13.8	12.4	16.4	13.7	12.3	16.3	13.6	12.2
35	16.5	13.8	12.4	16.4	13.7	12.3	16.3	13.6	12.2
36	16.6	13.8	12.4	16.5	13.7	12.3	16.4	13.6	12.2
37	16.6	13.8	12.4	16.5	13.7	12.3	16.4	13.6	12.2
38	16.6	13.8	12.4	16.5	13.7	12.3	16.4	13.6	12.2
39	16.7	13.9	12.5	16.6	13.8	12.4	16.5	13.7	12.3
40	16.7	13.9	12.5	16.6	13.8	12.4	16.5	13.7	12.3
41	16.7	13.9	12.5	16.6	13.8	12.4	16.6	13.7	12.3
42	16.8	13.9	12.5	16.7	13.8	12.4	16.6	13.8	12.3
43	16.8	14.0	12.5	16.7	13.9	12.4	16.6	13.8	12.4
44	16.8	14.0	12.5	16.8	13.9	12.5	16.7	13.8	12.4
45	16.9	14.0	12.6	16.8	13.9	12.5	16.7	13.8	12.4
46	16.9	14.0	12.6	16.8	13.9	12.5	16.7	13.9	12.4
47	17.0	14.0	12.6	16.9	14.0	12.5	16.8	13.9	12.4
48	17.0	14.1	12.6	16.9	14.0	12.5	16.8	13.9	12.4
49	17.0	14.1	12.6	17.0	14.0	12.5	16.9	13.9	12.5
50	17.1	14.1	12.6	17.0	14.0	12.6	16.9	14.0	12.5
51	17.1	14.1	12.6	17.0	14.1	12.6	17.0	14.0	12.5
52	17.1	14.1	12.6	17.1	14.1	12.6	17.0	14.0	12.5
53	17.2	14.1	12.6	17.1	14.1	12.6	17.0	14.0	12.5
54	17.2	14.2	12.6	17.2	14.1	12.6	17.1	14.0	12.5
55	17.2	14.2	12.6	17.2	14.1	12.6	17.1	14.1	12.5
56	17.3	14.2	12.6	17.2	14.1	12.6	17.2	14.1	12.5
57	17.3	14.2	12.6	17.3	14.1	12.6	17.2	14.1	12.5
58	17.3	14.2	12.6	17.3	14.2	12.6	17.3	14.1	12.5
59	17.4	14.2	12.6	17.3	14.2	12.6	17.3	14.1	12.5

Table A3.5 *WHO/NCHS normalized reference values for MUAC-for-length/height (65–145 cm)*

Length/ height[a] (cm)	Boys			Combined sexes			Girls		
	Median	−2SD	−3SD	Median	−2SD	−3SD	Median	−2SD	−3SD
65	14.6	12.7	11.7	14.3	12.4	11.5	14.0	12.1	11.2
65.5	14.7	12.7	11.8	14.4	12.5	11.5	14.1	12.2	11.2
66	14.7	12.8	11.8	14.5	12.5	11.6	14.2	12.3	11.3
66.5	14.8	12.8	11.8	14.5	12.6	11.6	14.3	12.3	11.3
67	14.9	12.9	11.9	14.6	12.6	11.6	14.4	12.4	11.4
67.5	14.9	12.9	11.9	14.7	12.7	11.7	14.4	12.4	11.4
68	15.0	12.9	11.9	14.7	12.7	11.7	14.5	12.5	11.5
68.5	15.0	13.0	12.0	14.8	12.8	11.7	14.6	12.6	11.5
69	15.1	13.0	12.0	14.9	12.8	11.8	14.7	12.6	11.6
69.5	15.1	13.0	12.0	14.9	12.8	11.8	14.7	12.7	11.6
70	15.1	13.1	12.0	15.0	12.9	11.8	14.8	12.7	11.7
70.5	15.2	13.1	12.0	15.0	12.9	11.9	14.8	12.8	11.7
71	15.2	13.1	12.1	15.1	13.0	11.9	14.9	12.8	11.7
71.5	15.3	13.1	12.1	15.1	13.0	11.9	15.0	12.8	11.8
72	15.3	13.2	12.1	15.2	13.0	12.0	15.0	12.9	11.8
72.5	15.3	13.2	12.1	15.2	13.1	12.0	15.1	12.9	11.8
73	15.4	13.2	12.1	15.2	13.1	12.0	15.1	13.0	11.9
73.5	15.4	13.2	12.2	15.3	13.1	12.0	15.2	13.0	11.9
74	15.4	13.3	12.2	15.3	13.1	12.1	15.2	13.0	11.9
74.5	15.5	13.3	12.2	15.4	13.2	12.1	15.2	13.1	12.0
75	15.5	13.3	12.2	15.4	13.2	12.1	15.3	13.1	12.0
75.5	15.5	13.3	12.2	15.4	13.2	12.1	15.3	13.1	12.0
76	15.6	13.4	12.2	15.5	13.3	12.2	15.4	13.2	12.1
76.5	15.6	13.4	12.3	15.5	13.3	12.2	15.4	13.2	12.1
77	15.6	13.4	12.3	15.5	13.3	12.2	15.4	13.2	12.1
77.5	15.6	13.4	12.3	15.6	13.3	12.2	15.5	13.3	12.1
78	15.7	13.4	12.3	15.6	13.4	12.2	15.5	13.3	12.2
78.5	15.7	13.4	12.3	15.6	13.4	12.3	15.6	13.3	12.2
79	15.7	13.5	12.3	15.6	13.4	12.3	15.6	13.3	12.2
79.5	15.7	13.5	12.4	15.7	13.4	12.3	15.6	13.4	12.2
80	15.8	13.5	12.4	15.7	13.4	12.3	15.6	13.4	12.3
80.5	15.8	13.5	12.4	15.7	13.5	12.3	15.7	13.4	12.3
81	15.8	13.5	12.4	15.8	13.5	12.4	15.7	13.4	12.3
81.5	15.8	13.6	12.4	15.8	13.5	12.4	15.7	13.5	12.3
82	15.9	13.6	12.4	15.8	13.5	12.4	15.8	13.5	12.3
82.5	15.9	13.6	12.5	15.8	13.6	12.4	15.8	13.5	12.4
83	15.9	13.6	12.5	15.9	13.6	12.4	15.8	13.5	12.4
83.5	15.9	13.6	12.5	15.9	13.6	12.5	15.8	13.6	12.4
84	15.9	13.7	12.5	15.9	13.6	12.5	15.9	13.6	12.4
84.5	16.0	13.7	12.5	15.9	13.6	12.5	15.9	13.6	12.5
85	16.0	13.7	12.5	15.9	13.6	12.5	15.9	13.6	12.5
85.5	16.0	13.7	12.6	16.0	13.7	12.5	15.9	13.6	12.5
86	16.0	13.7	12.6	16.0	13.7	12.5	15.9	13.7	12.5
86.5	16.0	13.7	12.6	16.0	13.7	12.6	16.0	13.7	12.5
87	16.1	13.8	12.6	16.0	13.7	12.6	16.0	13.7	12.5
87.5	16.1	13.8	12.6	16.0	13.7	12.6	16.0	13.7	12.6
88	16.1	13.8	12.6	16.1	13.8	12.6	16.0	13.7	12.6
88.5	16.1	13.8	12.7	16.1	13.8	12.6	16.1	13.8	12.6
89	16.1	13.8	12.7	16.1	13.8	12.7	16.1	13.8	12.6
89.5	16.2	13.9	12.7	16.1	13.8	12.7	16.1	13.8	12.7
90	16.2	13.9	12.7	16.2	13.9	12.7	16.1	13.8	12.7
90.5	16.2	13.9	12.8	16.2	13.9	12.7	16.2	13.8	12.7
91	16.2	13.9	12.8	16.2	13.9	12.7	16.2	13.9	12.7
91.5	16.3	14.0	12.8	16.2	13.9	12.8	16.2	13.9	12.7
92	16.3	14.0	12.8	16.3	13.9	12.8	16.2	13.9	12.8
92.5	16.3	14.0	12.9	16.3	14.0	12.8	16.2	13.9	12.8

Table A3.5 *(continued)*

Length/ height[a] (cm)	Boys			Combined sexes			Girls		
	Median	−2SD	−3SD	Median	−2SD	−3SD	Median	−2SD	−3SD
93	16.3	14.0	12.9	16.3	14.0	12.8	16.3	14.0	12.8
93.5	16.4	14.1	12.9	16.3	14.0	12.9	16.3	14.0	12.8
94	16.4	14.1	12.9	16.4	14.0	12.9	16.3	14.0	12.8
94.5	16.4	14.1	13.0	16.4	14.1	12.9	16.3	14.0	12.9
95	16.4	14.1	13.0	16.4	14.1	12.9	16.4	14.1	12.9
95.5	16.5	14.2	13.0	16.4	14.1	13.0	16.4	14.1	12.9
96	16.5	14.2	13.0	16.5	14.1	13.0	16.4	14.1	12.9
96.5	16.5	14.2	13.1	16.5	14.2	13.0	16.4	14.1	13.0
97	16.6	14.2	13.1	16.5	14.2	13.0	16.5	14.1	13.0
97.5	16.6	14.3	13.1	16.5	14.2	13.1	16.5	14.2	13.0
98	16.6	14.3	13.1	16.6	14.2	13.1	16.5	14.2	13.0
98.5	16.6	14.3	13.2	16.6	14.3	13.1	16.5	14.2	13.1
99	16.7	14.3	13.2	16.6	14.3	13.1	16.6	14.3	13.1
99.5	16.7	14.4	13.2	16.6	14.3	13.2	16.6	14.3	13.1
100	16.7	14.4	13.2	16.7	14.4	13.2	16.6	14.3	13.1
100.5	16.8	14.4	13.3	16.7	14.4	13.2	16.7	14.3	13.2
101	16.8	14.5	13.3	16.7	14.4	13.2	16.7	14.4	13.2
101.5	16.8	14.5	13.3	16.8	14.4	13.3	16.7	14.4	13.2
102	16.9	14.5	13.4	16.8	14.5	13.3	16.7	14.4	13.2
102.5	16.9	14.6	13.4	16.8	14.5	13.3	16.8	14.4	13.3
103	16.9	14.6	13.4	16.9	14.5	13.4	16.8	14.5	13.3
103.5	16.9	14.6	13.4	16.9	14.6	13.4	16.8	14.5	13.3
104	17.0	14.6	13.5	16.9	14.6	13.4	16.9	14.5	13.4
104.5	17.0	14.7	13.5	17.0	14.6	13.4	16.9	14.6	13.4
105	17.0	14.7	13.5	17.0	14.6	13.5	16.9	14.6	13.4
105.5	17.1	14.7	13.6	17.0	14.7	13.5	17.0	14.6	13.4
106	17.1	14.8	13.6	17.1	14.7	13.5	17.0	14.6	13.5
106.5	17.1	14.8	13.6	17.1	14.7	13.6	17.0	14.7	13.5
107	17.2	14.8	13.6	17.1	14.8	13.6	17.1	14.7	13.5
107.5	17.2	14.8	13.7	17.2	14.8	13.6	17.1	14.7	13.6
108	17.3	14.9	13.7	17.2	14.8	13.6	17.1	14.8	13.6
108.5	17.3	14.9	13.7	17.2	14.9	13.7	17.2	14.8	13.6
109	17.3	14.9	13.7	17.3	14.9	13.7	17.2	14.8	13.6
109.5	17.4	15.0	13.8	17.3	14.9	13.7	17.3	14.9	13.7
110	17.4	15.0	13.8	17.4	15.0	13.8	17.3	14.9	13.7
110.5	17.4	15.0	13.8	17.4	15.0	13.8	17.3	14.9	13.7
111	17.5	15.1	13.9	17.4	15.0	13.8	17.4	15.0	13.8
111.5	17.5	15.1	13.9	17.5	15.0	13.8	17.4	15.0	13.8
112	17.5	15.1	13.9	17.5	15.1	13.9	17.5	15.0	13.8
112.5	17.6	15.1	13.9	17.6	15.1	13.9	17.5	15.1	13.9
113	17.6	15.2	14.0	17.6	15.1	13.9	17.6	15.1	13.9
113.5	17.7	15.2	14.0	17.6	15.2	14.0	17.6	15.2	13.9
114	17.7	15.2	14.0	17.7	15.2	14.0	17.7	15.2	14.0
114.5	17.7	15.3	14.0	17.7	15.2	14.0	17.7	15.2	14.0
115	17.8	15.3	14.0	17.8	15.3	14.0	17.8	15.3	14.0
115.5	17.8	15.3	14.1	17.8	15.3	14.1	17.8	15.3	14.1
116	17.9	15.4	14.1	17.9	15.3	14.1	17.9	15.3	14.1
116.5	17.9	15.4	14.1	17.9	15.4	14.1	17.9	15.4	14.1
117	18.0	15.4	14.1	18.0	15.4	14.1	18.0	15.4	14.1
117.5	18.0	15.4	14.2	18.0	15.4	14.2	18.0	15.5	14.2
118	18.0	15.5	14.2	18.1	15.5	14.2	18.1	15.5	14.2
118.5	18.1	15.5	14.2	18.1	15.5	14.2	18.1	15.5	14.2
119	18.1	15.5	14.2	18.2	15.6	14.3	18.2	15.6	14.3
119.5	18.2	15.6	14.2	18.2	15.6	14.3	18.2	15.6	14.3
120	18.2	15.6	14.3	18.3	15.6	14.3	18.3	15.7	14.3
120.5	18.3	15.6	14.3	18.3	15.7	14.3	18.4	15.7	14.4

***Table A3.5** (continued)*

Length/height[a] (cm)	Boys			Combined sexes			Girls		
	Median	−2SD	−3SD	Median	−2SD	−3SD	Median	−2SD	−3SD
121	18.3	15.6	14.3	18.4	15.7	14.4	18.4	15.7	14.4
121.5	18.4	15.7	14.3	18.4	15.7	14.4	18.5	15.8	14.4
122	18.4	15.7	14.3	18.5	15.8	14.4	18.5	15.8	14.5
122.5	18.5	15.7	14.4	18.5	15.8	14.4	18.6	15.9	14.5
123	18.5	15.8	14.4	18.6	15.8	14.5	18.7	15.9	14.5
123.5	18.6	15.8	14.4	18.6	15.9	14.5	18.7	16.0	14.6
124	18.6	15.8	14.4	18.7	15.9	14.5	18.8	16.0	14.6
124.5	18.7	15.8	14.4	18.8	15.9	14.5	18.9	16.1	14.6
125	18.7	15.9	14.5	18.8	16.0	14.6	18.9	16.1	14.7
125.5	18.8	15.9	14.5	18.9	16.0	14.6	19.0	16.1	14.7
126	18.8	15.9	14.5	19.0	16.1	14.6	19.1	16.2	14.7
126.5	18.9	16.0	14.5	19.0	16.1	14.6	19.2	16.2	14.8
127	18.9	16.0	14.5	19.1	16.1	14.7	19.2	16.3	14.8
127.5	19.0	16.0	14.5	19.2	16.2	14.7	19.3	16.3	14.8
128	19.1	16.1	14.6	19.2	16.2	14.7	19.4	16.4	14.9
128.5	19.1	16.1	14.6	19.3	16.3	14.7	19.5	16.4	14.9
129	19.2	16.1	14.6	19.4	16.3	14.8	19.5	16.5	14.9
129.5	19.3	16.2	14.6	19.4	16.3	14.8	19.6	16.5	15.0
130	19.3	16.2	14.6	19.5	16.4	14.8	19.7	16.6	15.0
130.5	19.4	16.2	14.6	19.6	16.4	14.9	19.8	16.6	15.1
131	19.5	16.3	14.7	19.7	16.5	14.9	19.9	16.7	15.1
131.5	19.5	16.3	14.7	19.8	16.5	14.9	20.0	16.7	15.1
132	19.6	16.3	14.7	19.8	16.6	14.9	20.1	16.8	15.2
132.5	19.7	16.4	14.7	19.9	16.6	15.0	20.2	16.8	15.2
133	19.8	16.4	14.7	20.0	16.7	15.0	20.2	16.9	15.2
133.5	19.8	16.5	14.8	20.1	16.7	15.0	20.3	17.0	15.3
134	19.9	16.5	14.8	20.2	16.8	15.0	20.4	17.0	15.3
134.5	20.0	16.5	14.8	20.3	16.8	15.1	20.5	17.1	15.3
135	20.1	16.6	14.8	20.4	16.9	15.1	20.6	17.1	15.4
135.5	20.2	16.6	14.9	20.5	16.9	15.1	20.7	17.2	15.4
136	20.3	16.7	14.9	20.6	17.0	15.2	20.8	17.2	15.5
136.5	20.4	16.7	14.9	20.7	17.0	15.2	20.9	17.3	15.5
137	20.5	16.8	14.9	20.8	17.1	15.2	21.1	17.4	15.5
137.5	20.5	16.8	15.0	20.9	17.1	15.3	21.2	17.4	15.6
138	20.7	16.9	15.0	21.0	17.2	15.3	21.3	17.5	15.6
138.5	20.8	16.9	15.0	21.1	17.2	15.3	21.4	17.6	15.7
139	20.9	17.0	15.0	21.2	17.3	15.4	21.5	17.6	15.7
139.5	21.0	17.0	15.1	21.3	17.4	15.4	21.6	17.7	15.7
140	21.1	17.1	15.1	21.4	17.4	15.4	21.7	17.8	15.8
140.5	21.2	17.2	15.2	21.5	17.5	15.5	21.9	17.8	15.8
141	21.3	17.2	15.2	21.7	17.6	15.5	22.0	17.9	15.9
141.5	21.5	17.3	15.2	21.8	17.6	15.6	22.1	18.0	15.9
142	21.6	17.4	15.3	21.9	17.7	15.6	22.2	18.0	15.9
142.5	21.7	17.5	15.3	22.0	17.8	15.7	22.4	18.1	16.0
143	21.9	17.5	15.4	22.2	17.9	15.7	22.5	18.2	16.0
143.5	22.0	17.6	15.4	22.3	17.9	15.8	22.7	18.3	16.1
144	22.1	17.7	15.5	22.5	18.0	15.8	22.8	18.4	16.1
144.5	22.3	17.8	15.5	22.6	18.1	15.9	22.9	18.4	16.2
145	22.4	17.9	15.6	22.8	18.2	15.9	23.1	18.5	16.2

[a] Length below 85 cm, height at or above 85 cm.

For adults aged 20–59 years, as indicated in Chapter 3, bod
— calculated as weight in kilograms divided by the square of
provides a measure of thinness or underweight. The propo
tion with low BMI that would define a public health problem
available resources for correcting the problem, the stability
and government priorities. About 3–5% of a healthy adul
BMI below 18.5, and the following classification of the pub
low BMI has been suggested on the basis of BMI distribution
worldwide:[1]

Low prevalence (warning sign, monitoring required):	5–9% of popula
Medium prevalence (poor situation):	10–19% of popu
High prevalence (serious situation):	20–39% of pop
Very high prevalence (critical situation):	≥40% of popu

This classification is somewhat arbitrary, but reflects th
many populations of developing countries and endeavours to take
eration the societal consequences of the functional impairments commonly associated with low BMI. The proportion of underweight adults in a community is commonly (but not necessarily) similar to that of underweight individuals as a whole. If the proportion of *all* underweight is much lower than that for children, it is probably that the group most affected by undernutrition is children; this is likely to be because of recurrent infections or poor infant feeding practices. If both adults and children are affected, an overall food shortage in the community is the most likely cause.

The internationally accepted cut-offs for various levels of underweight are given in Table A3.6. It should be noted that there is commonly some increase in BMI between the ages of 20 and 24 years, particularly in developing countries. It has been a common practice to extrapolate data collected on adults to the elderly, yet it is not known to what extent BMI in the elderly has the same significance, because of the age-related decrease in height.[1]

For adolescents (aged 10–18 years), a WHO Expert Committee has recommended BMI-for-age as the best indicator of thinness. However, rapid changes in somatic growth in adolescence, problems of dealing with variations in maturation rate, and the difficulties involved in separating normal variations from those associated with health risks have been deterrents to developing a body of scientific knowledge linking adolescent anthropometry with determinants and health outcomes.[2] When nutritional oedema exists, malnutrition should be diagnosed in this age group. For stunting or low height-for-age the cut-off value is <3rd percentile or below −2 SD of the median NCHS/WHO reference values.

[1] *Physical status: the use and interpretation of anthropometry. Report of a WHO Expert Committee.* Geneva, World Health Organization, 1995 (Technical Report Series, No. 854).

[2] de Onis M, Habicht J-P. Anthropometric reference data for international use: recommendations from a World Health Organization Expert Committee. *American journal of clinical nutrition*, 1996, 64:650–658.

Table A3.6 *Adult weights and heights corresponding to specified values of body mass index*

Height (cm)	**Body weight (kg)**		
	BMI 18.5 (minimum normal)	**BMI 17.0 (moderate thinness)**	**BMI 16.0 (severe thinness)**
140	36.2	33.3	31.4
141	36.8	33.8	31.8
142	37.3	34.3	32.3
143	37.8	34.8	32.7
144	38.4	35.3	33.2
145	38.9	35.7	33.6
146	39.4	36.2	34.1
147	40.0	36.7	34.6
148	40.5	37.2	35.0
149	41.1	37.7	35.5
150	41.6	38.2	36.0
151	42.2	38.8	36.5
152	42.7	39.3	37.0
153	43.3	39.8	37.5
154	43.9	40.3	37.9
155	44.4	40.8	38.4
156	45.0	41.4	38.9
157	45.6	41.9	39.4
158	46.2	42.4	39.9
159	46.8	43.0	40.4
160	47.4	43.5	41.0
161	48.0	44.1	41.5
162	48.3	44.6	42.0
163	49.2	45.2	42.5
164	49.8	45.7	43.0
165	50.4	46.3	43.6
166	51.0	46.8	44.1
167	51.6	47.4	44.6
168	52.2	48.0	45.2
169	52.8	48.6	45.7
170	53.5	49.1	46.2
171	54.1	49.7	46.8
172	54.7	50.3	47.3
173	55.4	50.9	47.9
174	56.0	51.5	48.4
175	56.7	52.1	49.0
176	57.3	52.7	49.6
177	58.0	53.3	50.1
178	58.6	53.9	50.7
179	59.3	54.5	51.3
180	59.9	55.1	51.9
181	60.6	55.7	52.4
182	61.3	56.3	53.0
183	62.0	57.0	53.6
184	62.6	57.6	54.2
185	63.3	58.2	54.8
186	64.0	58.8	55.5
187	64.7	59.5	56.0
188	65.4	60.1	56.6
189	66.1	60.7	57.1
190	66.8	61.4	57.8

Interpretation
BMI < 16.0 indicates severe thinness
BMI 16.0–16.99 indicates moderate thinness
BMI 17.0–18.49 indicates marginal thinness
BMI 18.5–24.99 is the normal range for an individual

Note: A normal range of population median BMI of 21–23 has been suggested (see *Obesity: preventing and managing the global epidemic. Report of a WHO Consultation on Obesity.* Geneva, World Health Organization, 1998; unpublished document WHO/NUT/NCD/98.1, available from Programme of Nutrition, World Health Organization, 1211 Geneva 27, Switzerland.)

Body measurement techniques

Responsible personnel should be trained to measure and record weight, height, and/or arm circumference as described in the following paragraphs; see also Figs A3.1–A3.4 and the accompanying instructions.

Weight

Weight should be measured to the nearest 100 g (0.1 kg). Although various types of scales are used for weighing infants in the field, the most commonly used is the hanging spring balance scale, which can weigh up to 25 kg (see Fig. A3.1). The scale is hung from a branch, beam, tripod or — in the absence of other possibilities — from a pole supported on the shoulders of two adults. The infant is suspended from the scale in the specially designed pants or in a basket or sling, depending on local custom. If a basket or sling is used, the scale must be recalibrated to zero to adjust for the greater weight of the container.

Hanging scales of this type are robust, cheap, and easy to carry. Beam balances may be acceptable alternatives, although they are less portable. Bathroom scales are too inaccurate for field assessments, and bar scales are too bulky for mobile teams and more difficult to handle because they are less stable.

Calibration of the scales should be checked immediately before, and during, each session, using the same two known weights; the scales should first be set at zero with the weighing pants or basket attached. Suitable items for the calibration process include a lump of metal or rock, a 5–10 kg standard weight, or 5–10 litres of water. Spring balance scales should be replaced whenever the springs are so stretched that readings are incorrect. More details of the weighing procedure are appended to Fig. A3.1.

If a beam balance with a tray is to be used, it is important to ensure that the child sits properly and is not holding on to another person or to the static part of

Weighing procedure

Note: If the parent or carer or other untrained person is acting as the assistant, the measurer should carry out the weighing *and* record the weight on the record form.

1. *Measurer or assistant:* Hang the scale from a tree branch, ceiling beam, tripod, or pole held by two people, using a rope if necessary, so that the scale is at eye level. Make sure that it is secure. Ask the parent or carer to undress the child.
2. *Measurer:* Attach a pair of weighing pants (or infant sling or basket) to the hook of the scale and adjust the scale to zero; then remove the pants.
3. *Measurer:* Put your arms through the leg holes of the weighing pants (if used) (arrow 1). While the parent or carer holds the child, grasp the child's feet and pull his or her legs through the leg holes (arrow 2); make certain that the strap of the pants is in front of the child.
4. *Measurer:* Attach the strap of the pants to the hook of the scale. *Do not carry the child by the strap alone.* Gently lower the child and allow him or her to hang free (arrow 3).
5. *Assistant:* Stand behind and to one side of the measurer ready to record the weight (arrow 4). Have the record form and a pencil ready to hand.
6. *Measurer or assistant:* Check the child's position; make sure he or she is hanging free and not touching anything.
7. *Measurer:* Hold the scale and read the weight to the nearest completed 0.1 kg (arrow 5). Call out the measurement when the child is still and *the scale needle has stopped moving*; even the most active child will eventually become still long enough for a reading to be taken.
8. *Assistant:* Immediately record the weight and show your record to the measurer.
9. *Measurer:* Take hold of the child in one arm and gently lift him or her; release the strap from the hook of the scale with your free hand. *Do not lift the child by the strap of the weighing pants.*
10. *Measurer:* Check the recorded weight on the form for accuracy and legibility. If there are any errors, instruct the assistant to erase and correct them.

***Fig. A3.1 Use of the hanging spring balance for weighing infants*[1]**

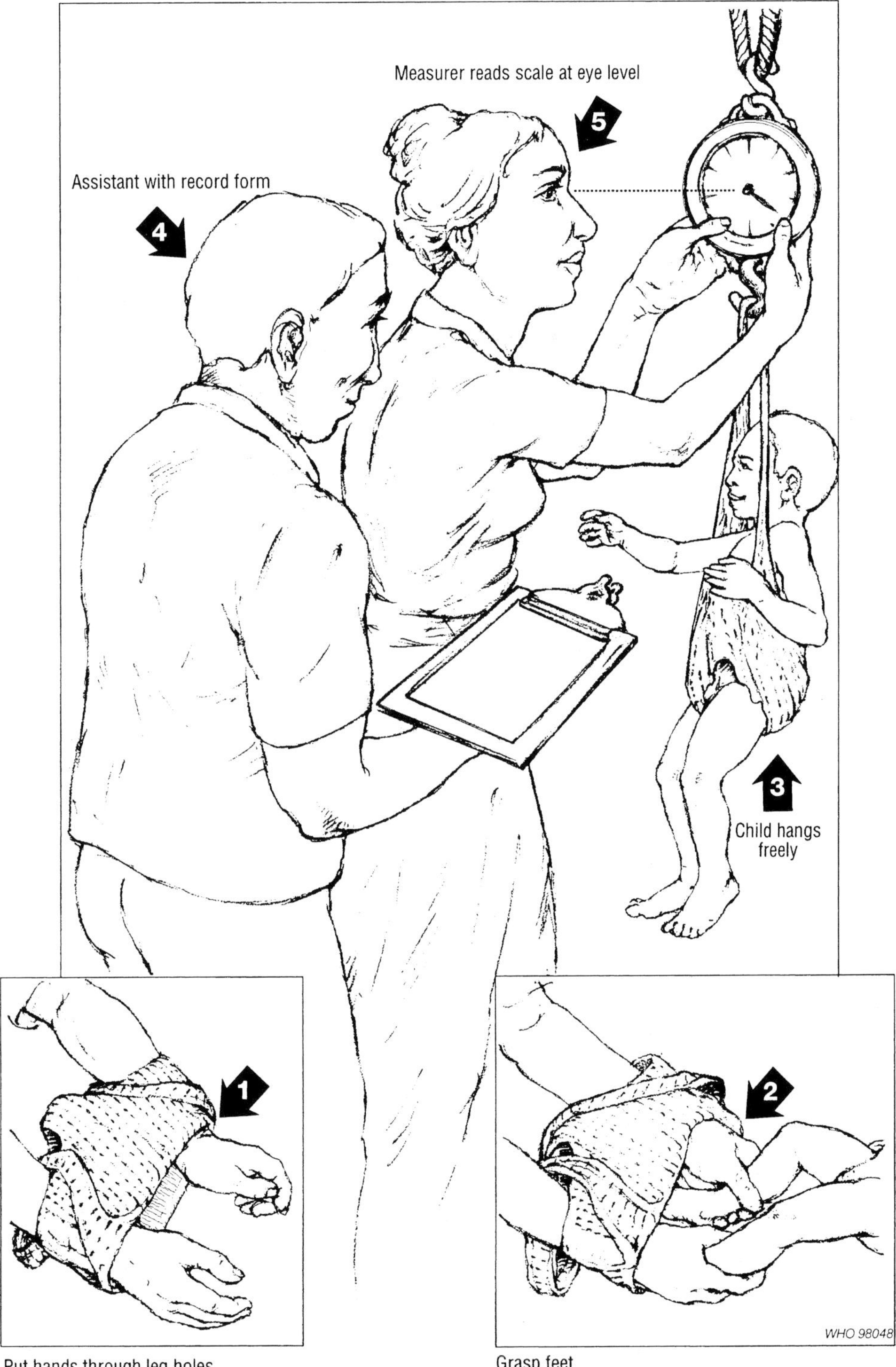

[1] Adapted, with permission, from *Assessing the nutritional status of young children: preliminary version.* New York, United Nations Department of Technical Co-operation for Development and Statistical Office, 1990.

the balance. A beam balance should be placed on a stable, horizontal surface, such as a wide board or a table.

Height or length

Every effort should be made to measure children's height or length accurately, to the nearest 0.1 cm if possible. Measurement errors of 2–3 cm can easily occur and cause significant errors in classifying nutritional status. Shoes and other footwear should be removed before measurements are made.

Length. A child under 2 years old or shorter than 80 cm (or 85 cm in a population that is *not* chronically undernourished) should be measured lying on its back. The child should be quiet, relaxed, and lying straight, with the head resting against a fixed head-board; the child should be looking vertically upwards. The help of the child's parent or carer is often valuable. Using one hand, the measurer should keep the legs straight by applying gentle pressure to both knees of the child and ensure that the movable slide is in contact with the surface of the soles and heels of the child's feet (not just the toes). More details of the procedure are appended to Fig. A3.2.

Height. A child over 2 years old (or taller than 80 or 85 cm) should normally stand to be measured. The child's heels should be together, at the back of the fixed foot-board. The buttocks, the backs of the heels, the upper back, and the head should touch the measuring board, which should have a metal tape-measure attached. The child's knees should not be bent. The movable head-board, which must be horizontal, should be slowly lowered until it rests firmly on the crown of the head (not just lightly on the hair). The vertical tape-measure is read opposite the highest point of the head when the child is looking straight ahead. More details of the procedure are appended to Fig. A3.3.

Measuring procedure

Note: If the parent or carer or other untrained person is acting as the assistant, the measurer should carry out *and* record the measurement.

1. *Measurer or assistant:* Place the measuring board on a hard, flat surface, e.g. the ground or a steady table.
2. *Assistant:* Place the record form and a pencil on the ground, close to hand (arrow 1). If the measuring board is on the floor or the ground, kneel down with both knees behind the base of the board (arrow 2).
3. *Measurer:* Kneel on the child's right side so that you can hold the foot-piece of the measuring board with your right hand (arrow 3).
4. With the help of the child's parent or carer:
   Assistant: Support the back of the child's head with your hands and gradually lower the child onto the board.
   Measurer: Support the child's body at the trunk.
5. *Measurer or assistant:* If the parent/carer is not also acting as your assistant, ask him or her to kneel on the opposite side of the board, facing you, to help keep the child calm.
6. *Assistant:* Cup your hands over the child's ears (arrow 4). With your arms comfortably straight (arrow 5), place the child's head against the base of the head-board so that the child is looking straight up. The child's line of sight should be perpendicular to the ground (arrow 6). Your head should be directly above the child's head. Look directly into the child's eyes.
7. *Measurer:* Make sure the child is lying flat, in the middle of the board (arrows 7). Place your left hand on the child's knees (arrow 8) and press them firmly against the board. With your right hand place the foot-piece firmly against the child's heels (arrow 9); the soles of the feet should be exactly vertical.
8. *Measurer and assistant:* Check the child's position (arrows 1–9) and correct if necessary.
9. *Measurer:* When the child's position is correct, take the measurement of length to the nearest completed 0.5 cm and call out the result to the assistant. Remove the foot-piece, release your left hand from the child's knees and support the child while the measurement is being recorded.
10. *Assistant:* Immediately release the child's head, record the measurement and show the record form to the measurer.
11. *Measurer:* Check the recorded measurement for accuracy and legibility. If there are any errors, instruct the assistant to erase and correct them.

A height arch can be used for selecting children shorter than 100 cm (or 110 cm in a population that is *not* chronically undernourished). This can be constructed simply, and should consist of a horizontal bar fixed 100 cm above the ground at right-angles to a vertical pole (or between two vertical poles). Any child who can walk under this horizontal bar without hitting it and without stooping should be referred (or included in the sample) for further measuring.

Arm circumference

Arm circumference is measured on the upper left arm. To locate the correct point for measurement, the child's elbow is flexed to 90°, with the palm facing up-

Fig. A3.2 Measuring a child's length[1]

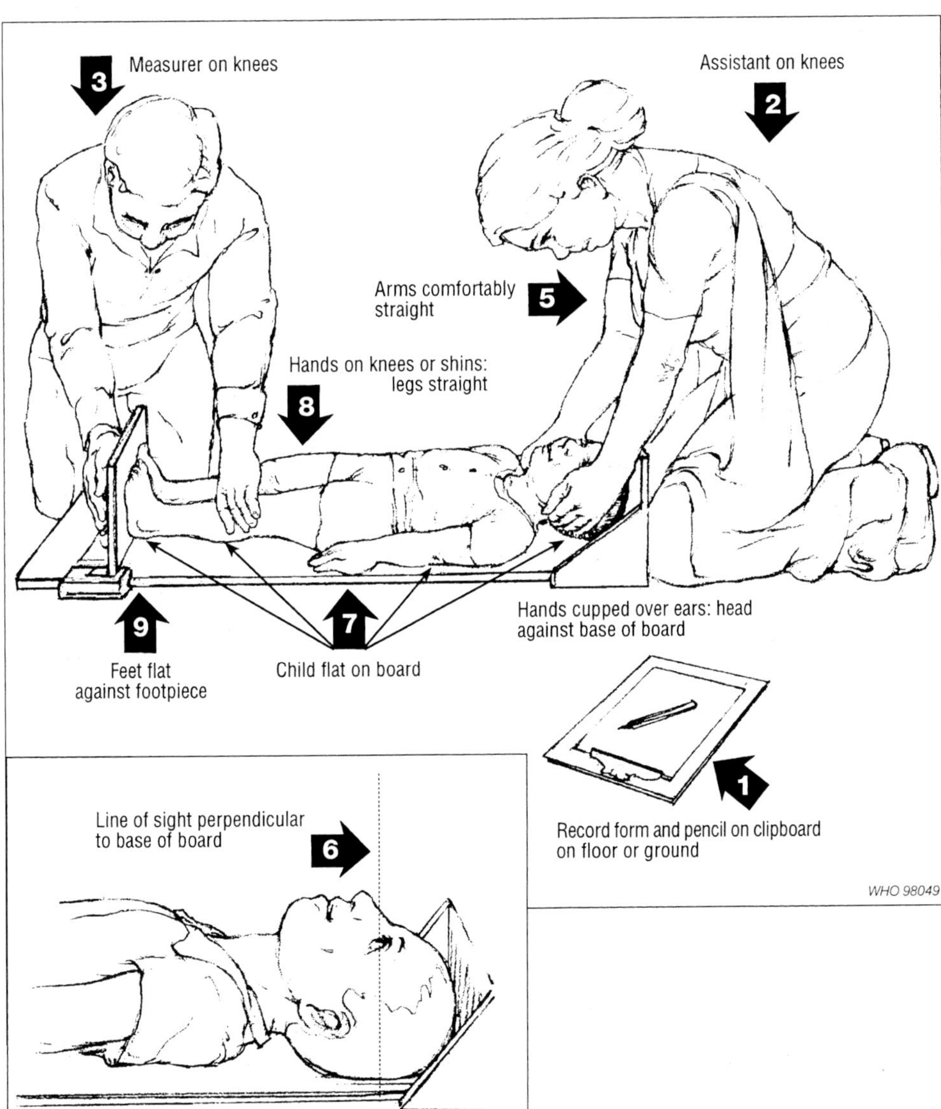

[1] Adapted, with permission, from *Assessing the nutritional status of young children: preliminary version.* New York, United Nations Department of Technical Co-operation for Development and Statistical Office, 1990.

Fig. A3.3 Measuring a child's height[1]

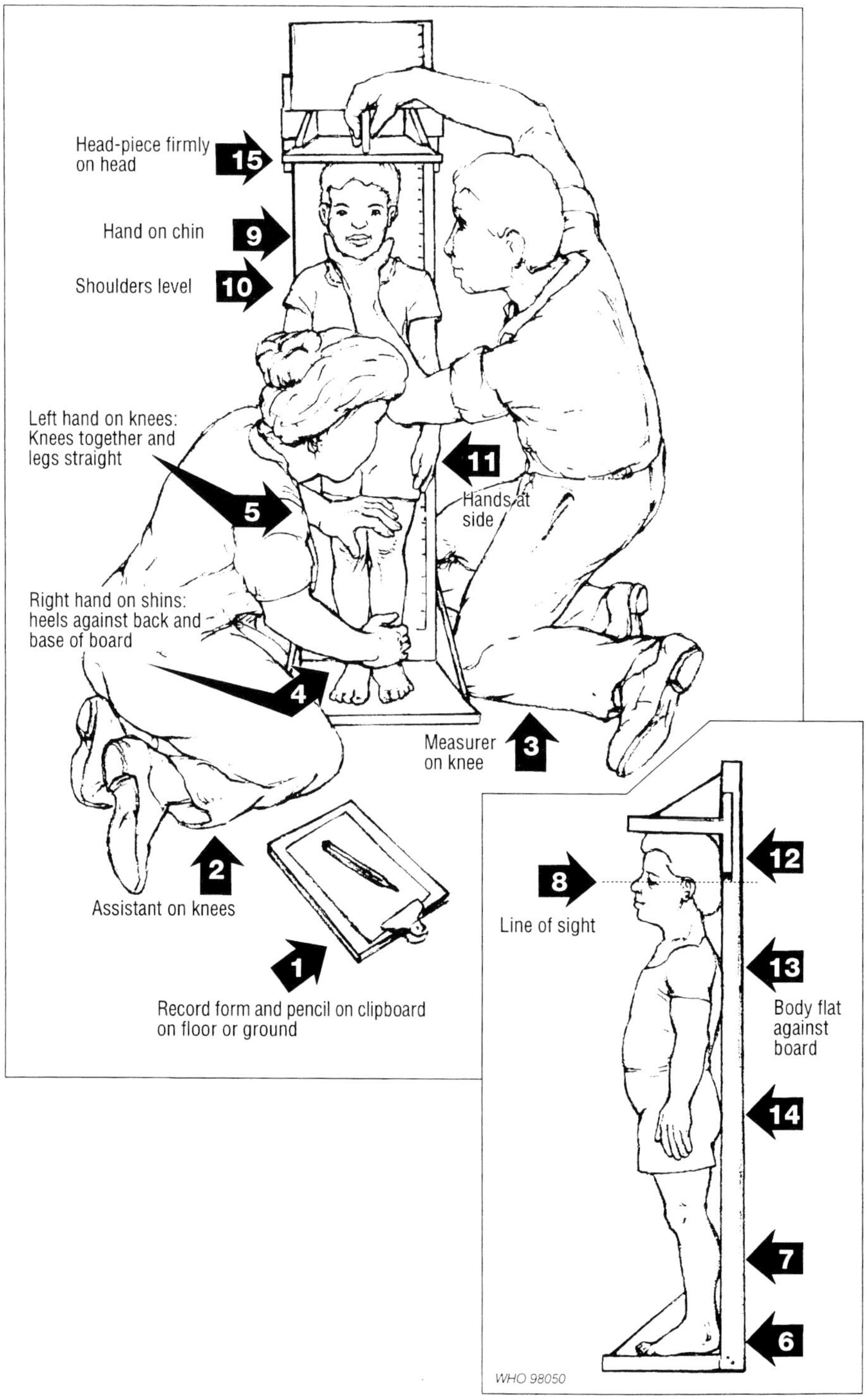

[1] Adapted, with permission, from *Assessing the nutritional status of young children: preliminary version.* New York, United Nations Department of Technical Co-operation for Development and Statistical Office, 1990.

wards. A measuring tape is used to find the midpoint between the end of the shoulder (acromion) and the tip of the elbow (olecranon); this point should be marked. The arm is then allowed to hang freely, palm towards the thigh, and the measuring tape is placed snugly around the arm at the midpoint mark. The tape should not be pulled too tight. Further details of the procedure are appended to Fig. A3.4.

For rapid assessment of nutritional status, the measured arm circumference can be related to a child's height by use of a special measuring stick — the WHO-modified QUAC stick.

Construction and use of the modified QUAC stick. To construct A QUAC stick like that illustrated in Fig. A3.5, use a piece of wood about 150 cm long and 3 × 3 cm in cross-section. On one face mark each 0.5 cm, from 0 at the bottom to, say, 145 cm near the top; write on it length/height for each full cm. On an adjacent face, mark the corresponding reference values for median −2 SD of MUAC-for-height (Table A3.5). Two sticks are preferable, one for boys and one for girls; otherwise, enter the values for the sexes combined. On the other face adjacent to the height markings, enter the values for median−3 SD of MUAC-for-height. Place the stick firmly and uprightly on a platform against a vertical wall. First measure the arm circumference as described in Fig. A3.4. Then have the child stand straight with his or her back flat against the stick and measure the height using a flat head-board. Note whether the arm circumference is less than that given on the "median−3 SD" face; if below it, record as severe deficit, and if above it, look on the "median −2 SD" face. If the measurement is below this value, record as moderate deficit; if above it, record as no deficit. All children can be identified in this way as having severe, moderate, or no deficit.

◄

Measuring procedure

Note: If the parent or carer or other untrained person is acting as the assistant, the measurer should carry out *and* record the measurement.

1. *Measurer or assistant:* Place the measuring board against a hard, flat surface, such as a wall, table, or tree, and make sure it is stable.
2. *Measurer or assistant:* Ask the child's parent or carer to remove the child's shoes, remove ribbons, and undo topknots etc. from the child's hair if these would interfere with measurement, walk the child to the board, and — if not acting as the assistant — kneel down in front of the child.
3. *Assistant:* Place the record form and a pencil on the ground, close to hand (arrow 1). Kneel with both knees on the child's right side (arrow 2).
4. *Measurer:* Kneel (on one knee only, for maximum stability) on the child's left side (arrow 3).
5. *Assistant:* Place the child's feet flat and together in the centre of and against the back and base of the board. Place your right hand on the child's shins, just above the ankles (arrow 4), your left hand on the child's knees (arrow 5) and push against the board. Make sure that the child's legs are straight and that the heels and calves are against the board (arrows 6 and 7). Tell the measurer when you have completed the positioning of feet and legs.
6. *Measurer:* Tell the child to look straight ahead at the parent or carer; make sure the child's line of sight is parallel with the ground (arrow 8). Place your open left hand on the child's chin and gradually close your hand (arrow 9). Do not cover the child's mouth or ears. Make sure the child has shoulders level (arrow 10), hands at the side (arrow 11), and head, shoulders, buttocks, and heels against the board (arrows 12, 13, 14). With your right hand, lower the head-piece on to the top of the child's head, making sure that you flatten the hair to the head (arrow 15).
7. *Measurer and assistant:* Check the child's position (arrows 1–15) and correct if necessary.
8. *Measurer:* When the child's position is correct, read and call out the measurement to the nearest completed 0.5 cm. Remove the head-piece from the child's head and your left hand from the child's chin; support the child while the measurement is recorded.
9. *Assistant:* Record the measurement and show the record form to the measurer.
10. *Measurer:* Check the recorded measurement for accuracy and legibility. If there are any errors, instruct the assistant to erase and correct them.

Fig. A3.4 Measuring child's mid-upper-arm circumference[1]

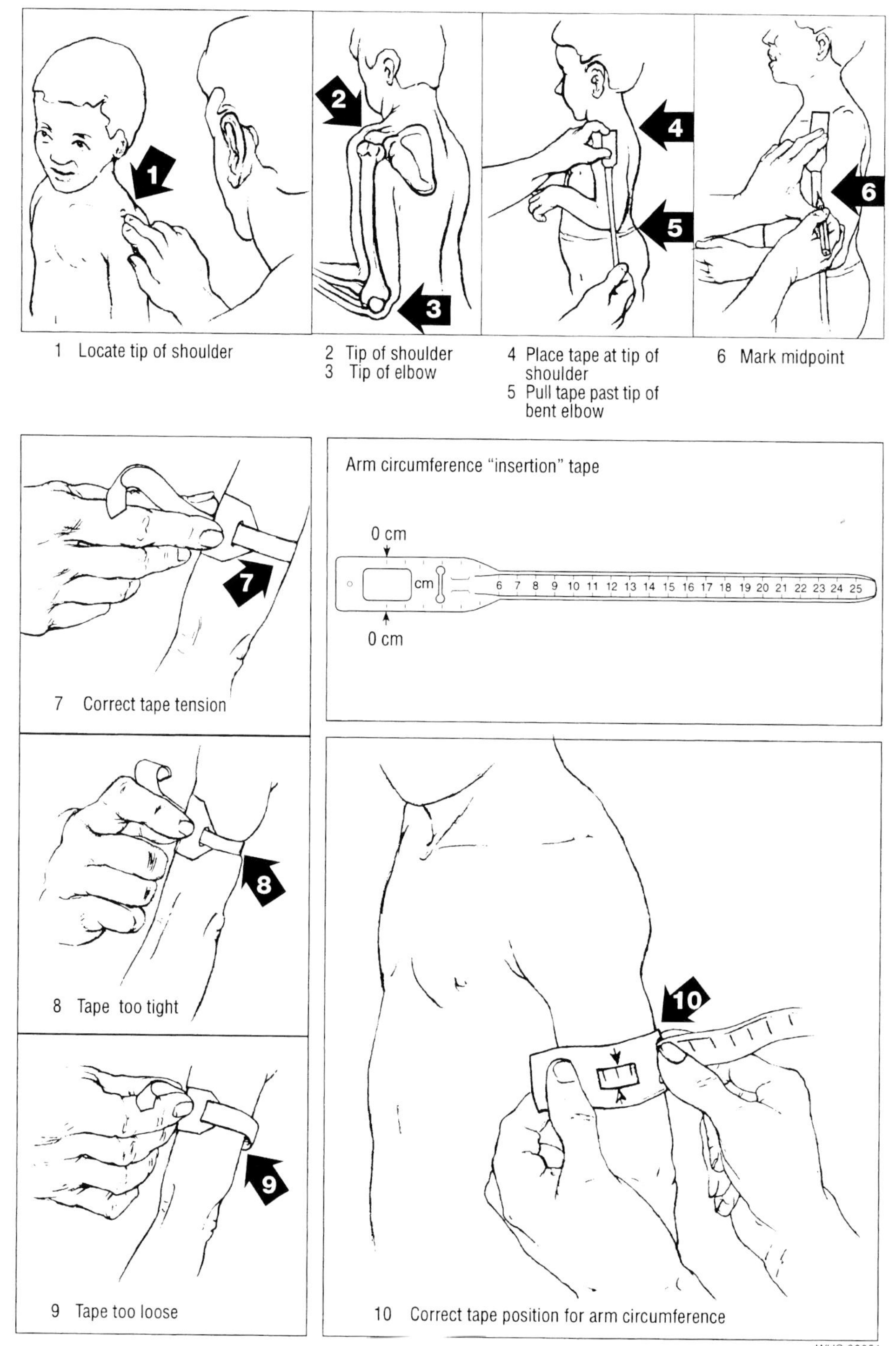

[1] Adapted, with permission, from *Assessing the nutritional status of young children: preliminary version.* New York, United National Department of Technical Co-operation for Development and Statistical Office, 1990.

Measuring procedure

Note: If the parent or carer or other untrained person is acting as the assistant, the measurer should carry out *and* record the measurement.

1. *Measurer:* Keep your work at eye-level and sit down when possible. A very young child can be held during the procedure by the parent or carer, who should also remove any clothing that covers the child's left arm.
2. *Measurer:* Calculate the midpoint of the left upper arm by first locating the tip of the child's shoulder (arrows 1 and 2) with your fingertips. Bend the child's elbow to make a right angle (arrow 3). Place a measuring tape at zero (indicated by two arrows) on the tip of the shoulder (arrow 4) and pull it straight down past the tip of the elbow (arrow 5); read the number at the tip of the elbow to the nearest 1 cm. Divide this number by 2 to find the midpoint, which you or your assistant should mark on the arm with a pen (arrow 6).
3. *Measurer:* Straighten the child's arm and wrap the measuring tape around the arm at the midpoint (ensuring that the numbers are right-side up). Make sure the tape is flat against the skin (arrow 7).
4. *Measurer and assistant:* Check that the tape around the child's arm is neither too tight nor too loose (arrows 8 and 9); correct if necessary.
5. *Assistant:* Make sure that the record form is ready and to hand.
6. *Measurer:* When the tape is correctly positioned and under the correct tension, read the measurement to the nearest 0.1 cm and call it out to your assistant.
7. *Assistant:* Immediately record the measurement.
8. *Measurer:* While the assistant records the measurement, loosen the tape from the child's arm.
9. *Measurer:* Check the recorded measurement for accuracy and legibility. Instruct the assistant to erase any errors and correct them.
10. *Measurer:* Remove the tape from the child's arm.

Fig. A3.5 The WHO-modified QUAC stick

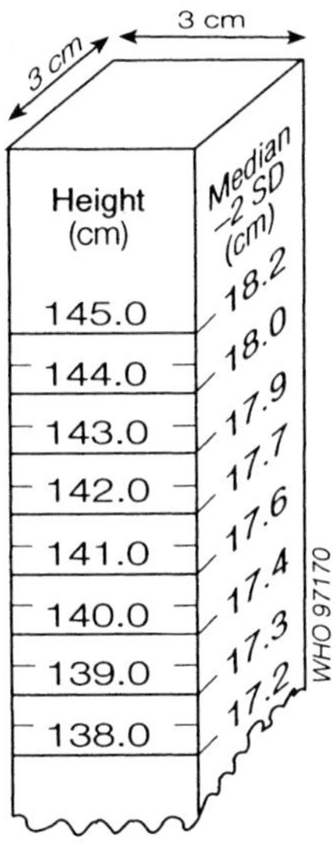

ANNEX 4

Statistical procedures for nutritional surveys

Introduction

This annex provides guidelines for statistical procedures, including sampling methods and determination of sample size, to be used in nutritional surveys. It fulfils the need — unmet by most handbooks, which deal more with surveys of communicable diseases — for guidance on the type of community-based survey essential for nutritional assessment.

The essential procedures for anthropometric surveys are covered in Chapter 3 and Annex 3; Chapter 2 outlines the parameters and criteria (mostly clinical and biochemical) used in assessing micronutrient deficiencies. In practice, a survey that combines clinical, anthropometric, and biochemical elements is required. Different types of nutrient are usually assessed in different age groups or among individuals of different physiological status, and few manuals provide guidance on how such assessments should be combined or integrated. Table A4.1 shows the suggested age/sex groups to be examined — usually on the basis of the household-selection procedure described in this annex.

Involvement of a statistician right at the start of the survey design process is important, to ensure that sample sizes are appropriate (neither too large nor too small) and will produce results from which valid comparisons can be made between different populations and in the same population over time. The sample size is usually similar for anthropometry and for assessment of the different types of nutrient, but the design factor (increase in size of cluster sample required because of patchy distribution of the deficiency) is generally recommended to be larger for micronutrient surveys (3) than for anthropometric surveys (2).

The first part of the annex deals with the principles of random sampling and with sample size, and the second part presents various sampling procedures.

Principles of random sample surveys

Basic concepts

When dealing with large population groups it is not feasible to survey all individuals. However, valid conclusions can be drawn from measurements made on only a limited number of individuals within the population, provided that this "sample" is representative of the population as a whole.

The sampling techniques described in this annex are designed to ensure this essential representativeness through randomization in selection and elimination of observer bias. Data obtained only from health services, for example, are

Table A4.1 *Examples of appropriate age/sex groups for nutritional assessments*

Age/sex group	Type of assessment
Children <5 years	Anthropometry Anaemia, vitamin A deficiency, beriberi, scurvy (if any cases seen)
Children of school age (6–12 years) and adolescents	Goitre prevalence; urinary iodine; anaemia/iron deficiency
Women of reproductive age, or pregnant women	Anaemia/iron deficiency, beriberi, scurvy
Adults	Anthropometry Beriberi, pellagra, scurvy (if any cases seen)

unlikely to be representative of the population as a whole; data collected only in the most accessible villages, or in camps that are reported to be in a bad state, will be similarly unrepresentative. Strict procedures must be followed in selecting individuals to be included in a sample to ensure that it is representative. Moreover, if the objective of a survey is to compare the nutritional status of two groups, representative data must be collected from the two groups separately.

The techniques, and the methods of analysing the results, recognize and allow for the fact that there may be some inaccuracy. Data gathered from a sample of a population provide only an estimate of what the results would be if measurements were made on the entire population. Whenever a sample is drawn, there is a risk that it may not be truly representative and therefore yield data that do not reflect the true situation. Inevitably, therefore, if a second sample is drawn from the same population, slightly different results are likely be obtained.

From a sample it is possible to calculate not only an estimate of malnutrition (or other variable of interest) but also the *range* of values within which the actual rate of malnutrition in the entire population almost certainly lies. The confidence interval is strictly not symmetrical, but as the sample size increases it becomes more and more symmetrical. For example, the 95% confidence limits for a 10% estimate of malnutrition based on a randomly selected sample of 30 children are 2% and 26%. However the confidence limits for a 10% estimate based on a sample size of 2000 are 9% and 11%. See Table A4.3.

A 95% confidence level[1] is usually considered to be appropriate for nutritional surveys. The precision of the result and the size of the confidence interval depend on the sample size and the actual prevalence of malnutrition (or other variable of interest) in the population.

Basic sampling procedure

Three main sampling methods can be used — random, systematic, and cluster. Cluster sampling is the most widely used and often the only feasible method in emergencies involving large population groups. In all cases, estimates are required of the total population and of any subgroups to be distinguished within the total. The essential steps in obtaining a sample are as follows:

[1] A 95% confidence level represents an *error risk* of 5%, meaning that, out of 100 surveys, as many as 5 may give results that do not reflect the true situation purely by chance.

1. *Obtain available population data.* Census data and a list of all settlements in the area might be obtained from departments of planning, statistics, or malaria control, for example. If no data are available, as may be the case for refugees or displaced persons, a rough population estimate should be made by counting the dwellings and estimating the number of people in each dwelling.
2. *Divide the total population into groups relevant to the information to be collected.* In the case of camp populations, it may be desirable to distinguish between different camps, different sections of camps, or between long-term residents and new arrivals. Among rural populations it is generally appropriate to distinguish pastoralists (such as nomadic herders), subsistence farmers, and others (including artisans and traders). If different groups are not distinguished, the survey findings may be difficult to interpret.
3. *Choose the sampling methodology to be used.* The required precision should be identified and the necessary sample size determined accordingly.
4. *Select the households or individuals to be examined.* The relevant sampling procedures should be followed carefully.

Defining sample size

The sample size is the number of individuals to be included in the survey to "represent" each population of interest. The sample size required depends on the following factors:

- *Required precision and confidence level.* The greater the precision required, the larger the sample needed.
- *Expected prevalence of malnutrition* (or other variable being estimated). The smaller the expected proportion of people presenting malnutrition, the greater the size of the sample required for a particular level of precision.
- *Time and resources available.* The time, personnel, equipment, transport, and funds available for the survey may limit the number of individuals or households that can be visited.

In practice, selection of sample size almost always involves a trade-off between the ideal and the feasible. A sample that is too small gives results of limited precision and therefore of questionable usefulness. For example, a result of 10% wasting (below median −2 SD weight-for-height) in a sample of 100 children would give a confidence interval ranging from approximately 4% to 16% — a result that cannot be interpreted usefully. Beyond a certain level, however, increases in sample size produce only small improvements in precision but involve disproportionate increases in costs. The formulae for calculating sample size (n) are as follows

- *for simple random sampling*

$$n = \frac{1.96^2 \times (1 - p)}{p \times \varepsilon^2}$$

• *for cluster sampling*

$$n = \frac{k \times 1.96^2 \times (1 - p)}{p \times \varepsilon^2}$$

where:

n = sample size required
p = expected prevalence of malnutrition in the population; as the prevalence of malnutrition is not known before the survey is done, an estimate must be used — this is usually an experienced guess, or derived from a small pilot survey
ε = relative precision required
1.96 is a statistical parameter corresponding to the confidence level of 95% (an error risk of 5%).
k = "clustering" factor, or design factor, which is a measure of the clustering of the characteristic being measured.[1]

p and ε can be expressed either as percentages or as fractions of 1 (10% = 0.10), but must both be expressed in the same terms.

The sample size for a cluster survey is likely to be larger than that for a random sample for the same precision. This is because the units within a cluster tend to be similar in their characteristics. Poor (and therefore malnourished) people, for instance, are likely to be found living together in the same areas.

Example

Expected prevalence of malnutrition 15%: $p = 0.15$

Relative precision required (ε) 20% of the estimated prevalence

Design factor $k = 2$.

For random sampling:

$$n = \frac{1.96^2 \times 0.85}{0.15 \times 0.20^2} = 544$$

For cluster sampling:

$$n = \frac{2 \times 1.96^2 \times 0.85}{0.15 \times 0.20^2} = 1088$$

Table A4.2 shows the sample sizes required for particular levels of expected prevalence and required precision with a fixed error risk of 5%. To take another example, if the expected malnutrition rate is 15%, and a relative precision of 3% is required, a sample size of 24 188 obtained by *simple random sampling* will be needed. For *cluster samples*, the figures in Table A4.2 should be multiplied by the appropriate design factor for the "clustering" of the characteristic being measured within sample clusters.

Table A4.3 shows confidence intervals at the 95% level (5% error risk) corresponding to various sample sizes and observed rates when random sampling is

[1] According to studies analysed by CDC, the design factor k usually has a value of approximately 2 in anthropometric studies among children under 5 years of age, with 30 clusters.

Table A4.2 *Sample sizes for estimating a population proportion with specified relative precision (95% confidence level)*[a]

ϵ[c] \ P[b]	0.05	0.10	0.15	0.20	0.25	0.30	0.35	0.40	0.45	0.50	0.55	0.60	0.65	0.70	0.75	0.80	0.85	0.90	0.95
0.01	729904	345744	217691	153664	115248	89637	71344	57624	46953	38416	31431	25611	20686	16464	12805	9604	6779	4268	2022
0.02	182476	86436	54423	38416	28812	22409	17836	14406	11738	9604	7858	6403	5171	4116	3201	2401	1695	1067	505
0.03	81100	38416	24188	17074	12805	9960	7927	6403	5217	4268	3492	2846	2298	1829	1423	1067	753	474	225
0.04	45619	21609	13606	9604	7203	5602	4459	3602	2935	2401	1964	1601	1293	1029	800	600	424	267	126
0.05	29196	13830	8708	6147	4610	3585	2854	2305	1878	1537	1257	1024	827	659	512	384	271	171	81
0.06	20275	9604	6047	4268	3201	2490	1982	1601	1304	1067	873	711	575	457	356	267	188	119	56
0.07	14896	7056	4443	3136	2352	1829	1456	1176	958	784	641	523	422	336	261	196	138	87	41
0.08	11405	5402	3401	2401	1801	1401	1115	900	734	600	491	400	323	257	200	150	106	67	32
0.09	9011	4268	2688	1897	1423	1107	881	711	580	474	388	316	255	203	158	119	84	53	25
0.10	7299	3457	2177	1537	1152	896	713	576	470	384	314	256	207	165	128	96	68	43	20
0.15	3244	1537	968	683	512	398	317	256	209	171	140	114	92	73	57	43	30	19	9
0.20	1825	864	544	384	288	224	178	144	117	96	79	64	52	41	32	24	17	11	5
0.25	1168	553	348	246	184	143	114	92	75	61	50	41	33	26	20	15	11	7	—[d]
0.30	811	384	242	171	128	100	79	64	52	43	35	28	23	18	14	11	8	5	—[d]
0.35	596	282	178	125	94	73	58	47	38	31	26	21	17	13	10	8	6	—[d]	—[d]
0.40	456	216	136	96	72	56	45	36	29	24	20	16	13	10	8	6	—[d]	—[d]	—[d]
0.50	292	138	87	61	46	36	29	23	19	15	13	10	8	7	5	—[d]	—[d]	—[d]	—[d]

[a] $n = (Z_{1-\alpha/2})^2(1 - P)/\epsilon^2 P$, where $Z_{1-\alpha}$ represents the number of standard errors from the mean, and α is the significance level of a test.

[b] P = anticipated population proportion (prevalence).

[c] ϵ = relative precision.

[d] Sample size less than 5.

Table A4.3 *Confidence intervals at 95% probability level corresponding to various sample sizes and sample percentages*

Sample size	Percentage observed in sample					
	5%	**10%**	**20%**	**30%**	**40%**	**50%**
30	1–18	2–26	8–39	15–49	23–59	31–69
40	1–17	3–24	9–36	17–47	25–57	34–66
50	1–15	3–22	10–34	18–45	26–55	36–65
60	1–14	4–20	11–32	19–43	28–54	37–63
80	1–12	4–19	12–31	20–41	29–52	39–61
100	2–11	5–18	13–29	21–40	30–50	40–60
200	2–9	6–15	15–26	24–37	33–47	43–57
300	3–8	7–14	16–25	25–36	35–46	44–56
400	3–8	7–13	16–24	26–35	35–45	45–55
500	3–7	8–13	17–24	26–34	36–45	46–55
1000	4–7	8–12	18–23	27–33	37–43	47–53
2000	4–6	9–11	18–22	28–32	38–42	48–52

used. For cluster sampling, the sample sizes must be multiplied by the appropriate design factor to take into account the clustering of the characteristic being measured.

If, for example, the observed malnutrition rate is about 20%, a total sample size of 100 will make it possible to estimate the true rate somewhere between 13% and 29%, assuming random sampling. If greater accuracy is required, for instance 18–22%, a sample size of 2000 would be needed.

In nutrition surveys in emergencies, the expected prevalence of severe malnutrition usually ranges between 5% and 20%, and the precision must be defined accordingly; a relative precision of 20–25% is generally appropriate.

The size of the total population does not normally affect the size of the sample required. However, if the population is small and the calculated sample size turns out to be greater than 10% of the total population, a correcting factor (finite population factor) can be applied as follows:

$$n_f = \frac{n}{1+f}$$

where

n_f = adjusted sample size for small (finite) population

n = sample size for large (infinite) population (for example, as set out in Table A4.2)

N = population size

$f = n/N$.

Calculating results and confidence intervals

When results have been calculated, the corresponding confidence interval, d, should be calculated as follows and reported:

- *for random sampling*:

$$d = \frac{1.96 \times (1 - p)}{np}$$

- *for cluster sampling* the following formula can be used to give an approximate result:

$$d = \frac{k \times 1.96 \times (1 - p)}{np}$$

Using a random number table

A set of random numbers is presented in Table A4.4. Numbers can be read in any direction — from left to right, right to left, top to bottom, or bottom to top.

Table A4.4 *Random numbers*

13118	50901	57493	96647	46146	65512	97571	49679	92251	36599
81111	33653	61544	90072	61635	94254	98222	49594	99403	56952
07124	56894	00475	09815	05299	17082	80775	11320	98562	68957
55155	23168	83063	80324	51450	68094	71844	68302	49552	12682
46406	44641	45461	75174	33268	86032	40355	58288	05532	29419
10616	17092	76614	04950	67982	28515	16782	86129	44391	64449
38497	57435	46124	37302	10783	93043	06903	77158	49638	26211
83203	45840	75843	75843	74567	75971	97779	98047	68916	35038
19236	62703	12863	14452	72228	55022	07024	43615	74802	02110
79024	60592	93692	29737	09314	26191	52484	11588	14078	85947
76073	57252	52795	67673	62267	29552	68244	49280	58583	42190
50568	66590	38807	30061	26336	46147	04554	44562	72604	63031
11838	73906	55981	23668	22627	88438	96686	73645	81410	10942
57618	30523	16757	11956	58411	41647	67884	30084	14500	66958
61846	47265	09508	11030	10462	93922	17022	71031	07827	94722
60935	25351	11687	07679	73455	58617	24415	56921	88450	50471
63328	21749	74262	77143	55995	50707	91516	38002	60552	00634
75937	07127	11014	00738	46159	09866	87587	41648	36538	24398
11981	89485	54965	08300	67724	24919	65682	50101	45470	07232
12311	17067	42758	64557	46297	28414	93801	81180	12176	08536
45160	76932	00433	42228	73696	27478	65321	22979	30198	86708
26427	48280	53441	44543	95231	39939	09251	09755	26671	89392
54568	17774	95705	28018	26507	63504	98872	22449	56423	59133
80855	94883	08969	16949	86045	68398	46164	57147	35104	37262
96203	73918	77875	48444	08167	58460	87945	52145	20330	77172
91210	89152	93904	27666	51080	00487	12073	41639	28717	33909
37808	11431	03351	82979	96677	41588	17592	5111x	84657	25427
47738	40686	00948	46598	99095	67011	05786	05642	26282	97486
03255	71561	78549	15611	49097	58375	70087	10066	83530	26684
92658	11755	39005	72386	20601	49630	85266	78939	89931	99674
86040	48908	88153	05616	91381	88378	28263	34725	80739	15251
87806	60615	14520	04557	72939	71060	10650	58769	07497	00808
46138	03111	47053	89391	83636	05877	17980	63940	23003	23737
81514	46994	77869	72054	22819	89316	77195	20194	65043	27706
28419	60216	07640	80670	84427	98368	99656	10214	04023	39899
99109	64711	06962	56790	96313	54470	18568	04319	31680	39507
15045	85129	03531	06107	93785	38290	00911	68388	68686	53357
61398	94861	90462	09438	53920	59996	91957	39255	86563	20781
58455	18205	39389	18286	22994	78421	22241	04228	86679	47840
81025	70374	79493	39386	41707	57491	35647	43409	37182	73435

Numbers can be read off with any required total number of digits. The steps involved in using this, or any other, set of random numbers are:

1. Decide on the direction in which numbers will be read; e.g. left to right going down the page.
2. Specify the required number of digits. If a random number is required in the interval 0001 to 1342, 4 digits are needed (any of which may be zero).
3. Close your eyes and stick a pin (or other sharply pointed object) in the table. Read off the required number of digits in the direction chosen in step 1, starting with the first digit to the left of the point. If the resulting number falls within the required interval, use this number. If not, repeat the process until an eligible number is drawn or move to the next number.

Sampling methods

All sampling methods involve a highly ordered form of selection designed to eliminate observer bias; each can be adapted in various ways depending on the situation. The paragraphs that follow provide a general description of each method and how it can be applied.

In all cases, each selected individual, or every child under 5 years old belonging to each selected household, must be seen and (for an anthropometric survey) measured. The survey team, with the help of the community, must find the individuals concerned, wherever they are. If necessary, the team must return later to see and measure an individual missed on the first visit. No substitutions can be allowed and no one can be missed (unless they have died or left the community being surveyed).

Random sampling

Random sampling is the best method — when it can be used — since it is the only one that ensures representativeness. An up-to-date list of all individuals in the population is needed, with enough information to allow them to be located. Individuals are randomly drawn from the list using a random number table (see above and Table A4.4). For a nutritional survey the sample would be restricted to children aged 6–59 months or 65–110 cm in length or height.

In practice, a reliable population list is rarely available, and it is sometimes practical to use the following alternative procedure:

1. Go to the area and make a list of *all* households included in the area of interest.
2. Assign each household on the list an identification number.
3. Select the required number of households using a random number table. Otherwise, pick household identification numbers out of a hat or a large box. (If this type of selection is done in public, the community can see how households are selected.) A number corresponding to each household is written on a small piece of paper, which is placed in the hat or box. The pieces of paper are shuffled and the required number of papers are then picked out (blindly). The households selected in this way become the sample for the survey.

4. Visit all of these (and only these) households. No households may be excluded or substituted for any reason. In a nutritional survey, all children in the specified age group belonging to each selected household must be measured.

Systematic sampling

Systematic sampling eliminates the need for complete, up-to-date population registers, but requires:

- a reasonably accurate plan or map showing all households; and
- an orderly layout, or site plan, which makes it possible to go systematically through the whole site.

This technique has been used in well-organized refugee camps, where households are arranged in blocks and lines. The procedure is as follows:

1. Either list all households and assign each one an identification number, or trace a continuous route on the map, which passes in front of every household.
2. Calculate the number of households to be visited in order to obtain the required sample. If the required sample size is 544 and there are, on average, 15 children (aged 6–59 months) per 10 households, the number of households to be visited is 544/1.5 = 362.6, or 363 (*round up* to the nearest whole number in this calculation).
3. Calculate the "sampling interval" by dividing the total number of households by the number that must be visited. If the total number of households is 5000, and 363 are to be visited, the sampling interval is 5000/363 = 13.8, or 13 (*round down* to the nearest whole number in this calculation).
4. Select the first household to be visited within the first sampling interval at the beginning of the list (or route) by drawing a random number which is smaller than the sampling interval. If the number drawn is 7, start with the seventh house.
5. Select the next household by adding the sampling interval to the first household identification number (or counting that number of households along the prescribed route), e.g. 7 + 13 = 20.
6. Continue in this way (e.g. 7, 20, 33, 46, etc.) until the number of households required for the survey has been systematically selected.
7. Visit all of these (and only these) households. No selected household may be excluded or substituted for any reason.

Two-stage cluster sampling

Two-stage cluster sampling is used in large populations, when no register is available and households cannot be visited systematically. Sampling is done in two stages:

1. Clusters, or sampling sites, within the total population are selected randomly. (Clusters may be natural groupings such as villages or, in a camp, blocks of a

few houses. Where natural groupings do not exist, artificial clusters may be defined by imposing a grid on a map of the area.)

2. Within each selected cluster, an appropriate number of individuals or households are randomly selected.

This process is applied separately to each population of interest. For instance, if a comparison is to be made between two separate, large refugee camps, the same number of clusters must be surveyed in each camp.

The larger the number of clusters, the higher is the probability of good representativeness of the population under study. In practice, physical constraints will limit the number of subjects who can be conveniently studied in a cluster; 30 subjects may often be the maximum to which easy access is possible in a community. The number of clusters to be examined is then derived by dividing the desired sample size, as determined below, by 30. It should be remembered that the sample size for clusters is larger than that for simple random samples.

Stage 1: selecting the clusters

Where feasible, the population is divided into a large number of clusters (at least 100) containing similar numbers of people using administrative, physical, or geographical boundaries. For this purpose, a map and a list of all separate identifiable units will be needed. Well defined villages of similar size are examples of possible clusters. Larger villages can be divided into two or more clusters. In a refugee camp, existing or imposed "sections" can be used. These clusters are numbered and then, using a random number table or systematic sampling, 30 are selected.

Alternatively, and more usually, the following procedure can be used:

1. Prepare a list of all existing units or zones with their estimated populations. (A unit or zone may comprise a village, camp, defined neighbourhood, or "section" within a camp.)
2. Add two more columns. In the first, record the cumulative population figures obtained by adding the population of each unit or zone to the combined population of all the preceding units or zones on the list, as shown in Table A4.5.
3. Calculate the sampling interval by dividing the total population by the number of clusters required (30). For example, if the population is 18 600, the interval will be 18 600/30 = 620.
4. Using a random number table, obtain a number between 1 and the sampling interval to define the unit or zone where the first cluster will be drawn. In the example in Table A4.5, a random number of 510 places the first cluster in unit 1.
5. Add the sampling interval repeatedly to the original random number (e.g. 510, 1130, 1750, 2370 . . .) to locate additional clusters up to the required total of 30, as shown in Table A4.5. Note that large population units are likely to be assigned more than one cluster; small units (with populations less than the sampling interval) may have none.
6. Within each unit to which more than one cluster is assigned (e.g. unit 3 in Table A4.5) further sampling is undertaken to locate the required number of

Table A4.5 *Example of first stage of cluster sampling*

Geograhical units/zones	Estimated population	Cumulative population	Attributed numbers	Location of clusters
Unit 1	800	800	1–800	1
Unit 2	310	1110	801–1110	
Unit 3	1220	2330	1111–2330	2, 3
Unit 4	550	2880	2331–2880	4
etc ...	...	...	...	...
...	...	...	...	...
Total	18600	18600	18600	(30)

Note: See page opposite for an explanation.

clusters within the unit. Make a sketch map of the unit or zone and subdivide the whole into subunits of roughly equal population (or numbers of households), as illustrated in Fig. A4.1. Randomly select from these the required number of clusters using a random number table or by drawing numbers out of a hat.

Never change a sampling site because it is too remote or is close to a bigger and "worse affected" place that someone feels should be surveyed in preference to the randomly selected "unimportant" site.

Strictly speaking, clusters for nutritional surveys should be defined on the basis of the numbers of children aged 6–59 months. In most situations, the proportion of children is relatively uniform, and figures for the population as a whole can be used, as indicated above. However, if there are known to be wide variations in the proportion of children in the populations of different areas, the numbers of children aged 6–59 months should be estimated and used as a basis for defining clusters. On the other hand, where reliable population figures are not available, clusters may have to be defined on the basis of estimates of the numbers of households in different units or zones.

Stage 2: selecting individuals within each cluster

Once the survey team is on site, the required number of children (usually 30) can be selected by systematic sampling, as described above, if the site layout permits. Alternatively, a sketch map of the area should be drawn, the houses numbered, and households selected using a random number table. In many situations, neither of these methods is feasible and the following procedure is adopted:

1. Go to the centre of the selected unit or cluster.
2. Randomly choose a direction by spinning a pencil (pen, bottle) on the ground (or a flat surface) and noting the direction in which it points when it stops.
3. Walk in that direction from the centre to the outer perimeter of the unit or cluster, counting the number of households along this line.
4. Using a random number table, obtain a number between 1 and the number of households counted.
5. Go to the household indicated and examine all children belonging to that household (e.g. if the number is 5, go to the fifth household along the randomly chosen line).

Fig. A4.1 Division of a unit or zone for the selection of clusters

Note: In most cases a population will be divided into at least 100 clusters, of which 30 will be selected.

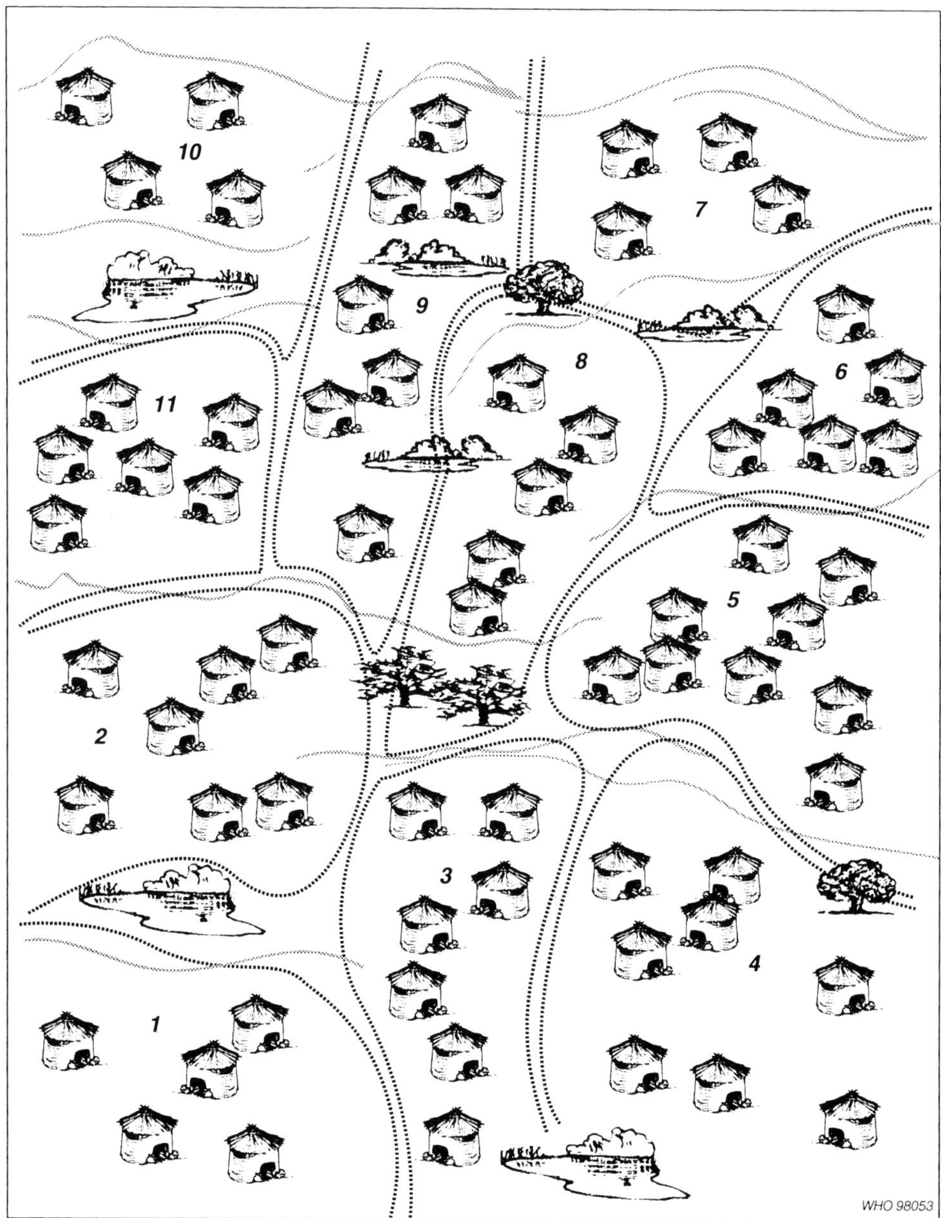

6. Go to the next nearest house, the one with the door nearest to the last house surveyed.
7. Continue the process until the required number of children (probably 30) has been completed.

The method to be used must be decided in advance and used consistently throughout the survey. It is important that there be no element of deliberate choice by the survey team in selecting the sample houses.

All children belonging to each selected household should be surveyed, including those in the last household (even if this means exceeding the number "required"). No substitutions can be made.

Thirty separate clusters should be surveyed if at all possible. If the number of clusters is reduced, the reliability of the estimate obtained may be poor and provide an inaccurate picture of the true nutritional status of the population being surveyed. A greater number of children per cluster does not compensate for a reduced number of clusters.[1]

[1] More than 30 clusters may be surveyed, but this will not significantly increase the accuracy or reliability of the results.

ANNEX 5

Use of particular foods in emergencies

Approximate nutritional values of some common food aid commodities

Table A5.1 summarizes the approximate amounts of nutritional energy, protein, and fat provided by 100g of various dry foods commonly supplied in food aid programmes.

Preparation of some food aid commodities

Small samples of food aid commodities should be cooked to make sure that recipes work; local cooks should be encouraged to experiment in preparing foods in traditional ways. Where necessary, local staff and recipients should be instructed in the best way to store and prepare foods to conserve the maximum nutrient content.

Bulgur wheat

Bulgur wheat and soy-fortified (SF) bulgur are provided as cracked whole grains, precooked to reduce cooking time and increase storage stability. These commodities should be cooked as follows:

- Add sufficient water to cover the grains in the pot. Proportions are about 1 part bulgur to 2 or 3 parts water. The volume of the grains more than doubles in cooking.
- If possible, soak for a few hours (overnight).
- Boil the cereals for 10–15 minutes in the same water (because B vitamins are present in this water). (Boil for 20 minutes if not soaked in advance.)
- Do not wash or rinse the grains after cooking.
- Pound finely (mash) for young children. (If the cereal is not cooked long enough, it is poorly digested by children.)

The same principles apply to most locally grown cereals.

Special blends

Corn–soy blend (CSB) and other blends can be used as dry ingredients, partially replacing cereal flours in many local dishes (breads, tortillas, chapatis, etc.). Depending on local cereal availability and acceptability, the proportion of CSB in a recipe can vary from 20% to 50%; oil and water content should sometimes be

Table A5.1 *Nutritional value of food aid commodities commonly used in emergencies*[a]

Commodity (100 g)	Energy ($kcal_{th}$)	Protein (g)	Fat (g)
Cereals			
Wheat	330	12.3	1.5
Rice	380	13.0	0.5
Sorghum/millet	335	11.0	3.0
Maize	350	10.0	4.0
Processed cereals			
Maize meal	360	9.0	3.5
Wheat flour	350	11.5	1.5
Bulgur wheat	350	11.0	1.5
Blended foods			
Corn–soy blend (CSB)	380	18.0	6.0
Wheat–soy blend (WSB)	370	20.0	6.0
Soy-fortified bulgur wheat	350	17.0	1.5
Soy-fortified maize meal	390	13.0	1.5
Soy-fortified wheat flour	360	16.0	1.3
Soy-fortified sorghum grits	360	16.0	1.0
Dairy products			
Dried skim milk (DSM) (enriched)	360	36.0	1.0
Dried skim milk (DSM) (plain)	360	37.0	1.0
Dried whole milk (DWM)	500	25.0	27.0
Canned cheese	355	22.5	28.0
Meat and fish			
Canned meat	220	21.0	15.0
Dried salted fish	270	47.0	7.5
Canned fish	305	22.0	24.0
Oils and fats			
Vegetable oil	885	—	100.0
Butter oil	860	—	98.0
Edible fat	900	—	100.0
Pulses			
Beans	335	20.0	1.2
Peas	335	22.0	1.4
Lentils	340	20.0	0.6
Miscellaneous			
Sugar	400	—	—
Dried fruit	270	4.0	0.5
Dates	245	2.0	0.5
Tea (black)	—	—	—
Iodized salt	—	—	—
High-energy biscuits	450	12.0	15.0

[a] Adapted, with permission, from *Food aid in emergencies*, Rome, World Food Programme, 1991.

increased. Alternatively, blends can be made into a porridge, which can be prepared as follows:

- Add CSB (or other blend) to water *while stirring*. If the mixture is lumpy, continue stirring until it becomes smooth.
- The porridge may be heated to boiling point, but should not be allowed to boil for more than 5 minutes to avoid destroying the vitamin content.

Whenever possible, oil should be added to the dry blend to increase the energy content, mixing and stirring thoroughly. The mixture (dry blend plus oil) can be stored for a few days in a dry place. After the addition of water and cooking, the blend should be consumed within a few hours.

Blended foods, e.g. CSB, are usually precooked and can, in principle, be added to *cold boiled* water and served immediately without cooking. However, great care is needed to ensure satisfactory hygiene and cooking is advisable for children under 3 years old. Blends must be made up freshly for each meal and be consumed quickly. (Blends can also be eaten in a dry form, or used to enrich a normal meal or a soup.)

Dried milks[1]

Dried skim milk (DSM) and dried whole milk (DWM) should be reconstituted by adding 1 part of dried milk to 4 parts of water, taking a small amount of *cold* water (1–2 parts), then slowly adding DSM or DWM, stirring until the solution is smooth. The remainder of the water can then be added (boil for 3–5 minutes if it is contaminated). If the dried milk is supplied in bulk, milk powder should be added to boiled cold water and whisked until the powder is well dissolved.

Dried milk can be added directly to porridge during preparation or before serving; it should be thoroughly stirred.

DSM is a major ingredient of the therapeutic liquid formulas (F-75 and F-100) used for treating severely malnourished individuals. See Chapter 5 for full descriptions.

Use of various food commodities

General principles

Foods to be distributed in relief programmes should be culturally appropriate, "rich" in the necessary nutrients, and appropriately packaged. Inappropriate or poorly packaged foods should be refused, returned, or destroyed.[2]

To the extent possible, relief rations should be made up of foods that the affected population is used to eating. This helps to ensure that food is not wasted, that tastes and food habits are not changed, and that dependency is not created. Special "relief" foods, including processed food aid commodities, are convenient to distribute and prepare, but they should *supplement*, not replace, traditional foods.

Suitable foods may be purchased locally where sufficient quantities are available, keeping in mind, however, that large-scale purchases may raise prices on the local market and cause hardship to the local population that buys its own food.

---

[1] See pages 200–203 concerning limitations in the use of dried milks.

[2] Some items offered to relief agencies are of intrinsically low nutritional value, e.g. soup mixes (because of the way they are used), some special foods for infants and young children, and other luxury foods. The nutrient content may be low or the water content high. Packaging is sometimes very bulky, e.g. for liquids, and this problem is aggravated if the product is packed in small unit volumes. The handling of such items wastes valuable fuel, finances, time, and other resources.

In situations where water and cooking fuel are scarce, commodities that require prolonged soaking (and discarding the water) or cooking should be avoided.

Food safety

Foods must be safe, i.e. *fit for human consumption*, both at the time of distribution and when they are consumed. When delivered, all commodities must have a sufficient shelf-life (in the prevailing storage conditions) to ensure that they will not have deteriorated or become chemically or microbiologically contaminated by the time they are distributed. Wherever possible, only those foods with a shelf-life of at least 6 months from the date of arrival in the country of distribution should be accepted. Imported commodities must conform to the food and sanitary regulations of the importing country.

A system of quality control should be implemented to ensure the safety and good quality of all foods distributed. Expiry dates should be checked, and foods should be inspected for signs of mould, rancidity, insects, or other deterioration or damage. If it is suspected that food has deteriorated during transport or storage, it should be tested by a competent authority (e.g. the public health laboratory) before it is distributed.

More details on food safety may be found in:

- *Hygiene in food service and mass catering establishment: important rules*. Geneva, World Health Organization, 1994 (unpublished document WHO/FNU/FOS/94.5, obtainable from Programme of Food Safety and Food Aid, World Health Organization, 1211 Geneva 27, Switzerland).

Packaging

All imported foods should arrive in packaging that is clearly labelled in an appropriate language with the following specifications:

- production date
- shelf-life and expiration date[1]
- actual contents and composition
- nutritive value.

Packaging should be strong enough to withstand rough handling and changes in temperature and humidity. At the same time it must be lightweight and easy to open.

Some commodities are best provided in large containers (e.g. cereals in 50-kg sacks), while others are more conveniently distributed in small containers (e.g. oil in 1-litre or 5-litre cans). However, small containers are susceptible to both damage and pilferage during transport, storage, and handling operations, and losses are sometimes very high. Donors should be advised at the earliest stage of the emergency about the most appropriate quantities and packaging, and about the suitability, quantity, and type of existing stocks.

---

[1] Shelf-life will vary with storage conditions.

Considerations relating to specific food items

Cereals

Cereals usually supply the bulk of energy requirements, plus a significant amount of protein. It is important to provide a cereal that is traditionally used by the population concerned and to distribute it in a form (whole grain or milled) that is familiar and can be easily used.

Cereal blends

Various cereal-based blended foods (in the form of flours) are available from international donors. Blends are also produced in some developing countries (e.g. "faffa" in Ethiopia and "likuni phala" in Malawi). Most are fortified with vitamins and minerals (labels should be checked) and many are used as complementary foods. Detailed guidelines on the nutritional and technical aspects of the production of formulated supplementary foods for small children are provided in Volume 4 of the Codex Alimentarius.[1] Examples of fortified blended foods are given in Table A5.2.

Fortified blends may be used for supplements for vulnerable groups, especially pregnant women, and as complementary foods during the weaning period. They are valuable in general rations as sources of vitamins and minerals when no fresh food items are available.

Most blended foods have the advantage of being quickly prepared with cold water since they are precooked. However, care must be taken to avoid their contamination during reconstitution, and it may not be possible to mobilize large quantities at short notice.

Table A5.2 *Micronutrient content of selected blended foods*[a]

Food	Micronutrient content per 100-g portion							
	Calcium (mg)	Iron (mg)	Vitamin A (mg)	Thiamine (mg)	Riboflavin (mg)	Niacin (mg)	Folate (μg)	Vitamin C (mg)
Corn–soy blend	513	18.5	500	0.65	0.50	6.8	U[b]	40
Wheat–soy blend	750	20.8	498	1.50	0.60	9.1	U[b]	40
Soy-fortified bulgur wheat	54	4.7	0	0.25	0.13	4.2	74	0
Soy-fortified cornmeal	178	4.8	228	0.70	0.30	3.1	U[b]	0
Soy-fortified wheat flour (11–12% soy)	211	4.8	265	0.66	0.36	4.6	U[b]	0
Soy-fortified sorghum grits	40	2.0	0	0.20	0.10	1.7	50	0

[a] Source: *Food and nutrition in the management of group feeding programmes*, Rev. 1. Rome, Food and Agriculture Organization of the United Nations, 1993

[b] U = no value could be found for the micronutrient.

[1] Codex Alimentarius Commission. *Codex Alimentarius. Vol. 4. Foods for special dietary uses (including foods for infants and children)*, 2nd ed. Rome, Food and Agriculture Organization of the United Nations, 1994:53–64.

Pulses

Pulses (or "legumes", e.g. beans, peas, lentils) are the most common protein-rich foods used in emergencies. They are easier to transport and distribute, and less likely to become contaminated, than meat or fish. As with cereals, every effort must be made to provide the most culturally acceptable variety, although local preferences should be weighed against the method of preparation, especially when water and fuel are limited. Many types of bean, for example, require cooking for as long as 4–5 hours if they are not soaked beforehand. When cooking fuel and water are scarce, pulses that take less time to cook (e.g. lentils or split peas) should be used.

Cooking oil

Any of the numerous vegetable oils that meet commercial standards is acceptable for emergency distribution. Palm oil has the best nutritional quality in this context since it is a very rich source of provitamin A; its provision is to be encouraged in populations accustomed to it. In general, animal fats should be avoided because of cultural sensitivities, although butter oil (or ghee) may be preferred in a few societies.

Salt

Salt is essential in the diet and may be a useful or necessary ingredient in emergency rations. It improves the taste of food and compensates for losses of this essential nutrient from the body, especially in hot climates. It is also needed for the preparation of oral rehydration solution at household level. Iodized salt should be provided in areas where iodine deficiency is endemic; it can usually be purchased locally or in a neighbouring country.

Sugar

Sugar may improve the taste of beverages and boosts the energy density of complementary weaning foods; it is also needed for home or on-site preparation of oral rehydration solution and for the preparation of therapeutic liquid diets. However, it is not wise to accustom children to eat only sweetened foods.

Meat and fish

Meat and fish are occasionally available and distributed in dried or tinned form. **Only those commodities that are culturally acceptable should be provided** (e.g. no pork for Muslim communities). If tinned products are used they should be 100% meat or fish, packed in oil or natural juices (not sauces or spices). Clear labelling of tins is essential and should include the expiration date. Tins should be packed compactly in strong cartons, which should also contain a sufficient number of appropriate openers.

Fish-protein concentrates

Fish-protein concentrates can be added to traditional dishes or consumed with no additional preparation, even by infants. They are a high-quality source of protein. However, the products should be field-tested among target beneficiaries before being ordered or distributed; the taste may be much enjoyed by some but thoroughly disliked by others.

Fruits and vegetables

Fresh fruits and vegetables are valuable sources of vitamins and minerals; they contribute both to the palatability of a meal and to the satisfaction derived from it. Where they are available from local markets, frequent purchases and distribution are necessary; the least perishable varieties should be used whenever possible. Dried fruits are relatively easy to distribute and should be used if they are available and acceptable. A good range of vegetables is essential to a well balanced diet.

Spices

Spices have no intrinsic nutritional value. However, they greatly enhance the taste of other (even unfamiliar) foods, and so encourage consumption and better nutrition. They are usually available for local purchase.

Tea and coffee

Where possible, tea or coffee should be made available, either through general distribution or through trading or payment (if appropriate). They have little nutritional value but may help to maintain social cohesion.

Honey, cheese, and nuts

Items such as honey, cheese, and nuts are occasionally offered by donors for relief distribution and may be appropriate in selective feeding programmes. They can be an incentive to ensure attendance at ration distribution points.

Biscuits

Only "high-energy" biscuits, which provide a minimum of 400 $kcal_{th}$ and 12 g of protein per 100 g, should be used in special feeding programmes. The biscuits should also be fortified with vitamins and minerals.

Milk products

See page 200.

Inappropriate foods for emergency feeding

Infant foods

Commercially prepared weaning foods are costly and unsuitable as relief items. If such items are required for exceptional cases, they should be provided through health facilities under strictly controlled conditions. Cereal blends, such as corn–soy blend, are suitable substitutes to use in preparing complementary foods. Breast-milk substitutes are discussed in Annex 6.

Confectionery or sweetened milk

Sweetened milks encourage poor eating habits and cause dental caries, especially in children. In particular, sweetened condensed milk is unsuitable for infant feeding. Confectionery is inappropriate and liquid preparations are heavy and thus expensive to transport and store.

Freeze-dried foods

Freeze-dried (lyophilized) foods pose no specific health risk and are very light to transport. They are nevertheless inappropriate for two reasons. First, they are almost certainly unfamiliar to, and therefore inappropriate for, those requiring emergency feeding. Second, their cost is prohibitive: a quantity sufficient to provide 100 $kcal_{th}$ costs at least 60 times as much as traditional foods. They should not be used as emergency relief supplies.

"Diet" (low-calorie or low-fat) products

Diet or slimming products are sometimes offered as "high-protein" foods. They are actually low-energy/high-bulk products and have no place in emergency feeding programmes.

Vitamin liquids or semi-liquids

So-called vitamin-enriched and/or mineral-enriched fluids are sometimes offered. They inevitably contain at least 90% water and are *never* appropriate for emergency feeding programmes.

Use of milk powder in relief operations

Milk powders are potentially valuable, concentrated sources of good-quality protein and other nutrients. However, since improperly prepared milk powder can be hazardous because of contamination and incorrect dilution, and its availability can discourage breast-feeding, the use of milk powders should be tightly controlled. **Milk powders should never be distributed alone as part of the general dry ration.** Nevertheless, milk powders can be used in the following circumstances:

(a) in well supervised supplementary and therapeutic feeding programmes for children aged 6 months and above, where proper care is taken to prepare the milk correctly and safely (see Chapters 4, 5, and 6);

(b) in orphanages, where on-site feeding is closely supervised and safe;

(c) in pastoral communities who traditionally use soured milk products and who can be taught how to prepare them from milk powders and use them safely;

(d) blended with cereals, and distributed as such (e.g. corn–soy milk), with proper instructions on their use for infants beyond 6 months of age and young children, or for vulnerable adults, e.g. pregnant women;

(e) where breast-feeding may be hazardous to the infant (because of tuberculosis, AIDS, etc.) and the mother, under regular supervision, has the resources, will, and skill to prepare safe and adequate artificial feeds (see Annex 6);

Table A5.3 *Nutritional value of dried milks*

	Energy ($kcal_{th}$) per 100 g	Protein (g) per 100 g	Fat (g) per 100 g	Vitamin A (IU) per 100 g
DSM(E)	360	36	1	5000
DWM	500	26	27	1200

(f) for other infants whose mothers have died or are unable to breast-feed (e.g. because of severely incapacitating mental disorder) and for whom wet-nurses cannot be found;

(g) in similarly supervised circumstances, for indviduals suffering from those extremely rare pathophysiological conditions in which breast-feeding cannot be effective (see Annex 6).

Breast-milk substitutes of adequate quality may justifiably be used in an emergency situation in categories (b), (e), (f), and (g) above, for infants under 6 months. An emergency situation does not of itself justify the use of breast-milk substitutes; the usual stringent criteria still apply. See Annex 6.

Various types of dried milk products are offered by food aid donors. The two main types are:

- Dried skim milk (DSM), which exists in two forms:
  - DSM(P) = DSM plain: contains no vitamin A
  - DSM(E) = DSM-enriched: fortified with vitamin A.

  Of these, *only DSM(E)* should be used in emergency feeding programmes, because all individuals in emergencies are likely to have low vitamin A stores and too little vitamin A in their daily diet.

- Dried whole milk (DWM), which contains fat and vitamin A. This is also referred to as dried full-cream milk (DFCM).

All personnel concerned should be made aware of the differences between these milk products and take great care when specifying requirements and issuing instructions to field staff. Any milk powder that is distributed should be in containers on which instructions for its correct and safe reconstitution are clearly marked. The instructions should be in an appropriate language and the simplest terms, e.g. 1 measure [specify measure] of milk powder mixed with x measures of water.

There are important differences between DSM(E) and DWM in terms of their nutritional value and reconstitution,[1] which are summarized in Table A5.3.

When it is appropriate to use milk as a beverage for selective on-site feeding, whole milk powder (containing approximately 25% fat) can be reconstituted by adding only safe water. Dried skim milk has had almost all its fat content removed and should thus be reconstituted with oil and water. Either product can be used in preparing a liquid diet for therapeutic or supplementary feeding, but

[1] There are also differences in cost. According to the World Food Programme, in 1991 DWM cost nearly 50% more per ton than DSM(E).

DSM is more cost-effective. In addition, DSM can be appropriately used in on-site feeding programmes to increase the protein content of meals by adding it *in dry form* to porridges and other foods.[1]

Storage

The shelf-life of powdered milk depends more on packaging than on the type of product. Most dried milk powder supplied by the World Food Programme can be stored for between 6 months and 2 years, depending on mean maximum daily temperature:[2]

- in a cold climate (4 °C) — 24 months
- in subtropical conditions (21 °C) — 12–18 months
- in a very warm climate (32 °C) — 6 months.

However, safe storage time varies also with storage conditions, especially humidity and possibility or extent of contamination. Packages of milk powder should carry labels indicating "Use before [date]" or equivalent guidance on storage conditions and shelf-life. No single rule is universally applicable.

Milk powder should be tasted to check for rancidity. If it causes an acid sensation in the mouth or throat, it is rancid.

Further details on food storage may be found in:

- Walker DJ, ed. *Food storage manual*. Rome, and Chatham, England, World Food Programme and Natural Resources Institute, 1992.

Principles for milk powder distribution

The policy of UNHCR relating to the acceptance, distribution, and use of milk products in refugee settings comprises the principles outlined below. It was developed in cooperation with WHO and has also been adopted by WFP.[3] It is appropriate for governments and other agencies as well. Apart from the above-mentioned exception regarding pastoralist communities (see item (c), page 200), these principles should be applied in respect of milk-powder distribution in all relief operations:

1. Accept, supply, and distribute donations of milk products only if they can be used under strict control and in hygienic conditions, e.g. in a supervised environment for on-the-spot consumption.
2. Accept, supply, and distribute milk products only when received in a dry form. Liquid or semi-liquid products including evaporated or condensed milk will not be accepted.

---

[1] In a few cases, donated DSM is mixed with a suitable cereal flour *before* delivery to distribution sites, or used as an ingredient in the local production of processed foods such as noodles (for general distribution) or biscuits (for supplementary feeding). This is consistent with the general statement on page 200.

[2] *Food aid in emergencies*. Rome, World Food Programme, 1991.

[3] These guidelines were issued by UNHCR in 1989 (Inter-Office Memorandum No. 88/89, Field Office Memorandum No. 76/89, 25 July 1989). "Milk products" includes any non-fresh milk product such as powdered, evaporated, condensed, or otherwise modified milk, including infant formula.

3. Accept, supply, and distribute dried milk (DSM) only if it has been fortified with vitamin A.
4. Support the principle that, in general feeding programmes, protein sources such as pulses, meat, or fish are preferred to dried skim milk. DSM premixed centrally with cereal flour and sugar is useful for feeding young children, especially if prepared with oil.
5. Advocate the distribution of dried milk in a take-away form only if it has been previously mixed with a suitable cereal flour, and only when culturally acceptable. The sole exception to this may be where milk forms an essential part of the traditional diet (e.g. among nomadic populations) and can be used safely.
6. Adopt the policy of the World Health Organization concerning safe and appropriate infant and young child feeding, in particular by protecting, promoting, and supporting breast-feeding, and encouraging the timely and correct use of complementary foods in refugee settings.
7. Discourage the distribution and use of breast-milk substitutes in refugee settings. When such substitutes are absolutely necessary, they will be provided together with clear instructions for safe mixing and for feeding with a cup, and with a warning as to their dangers.
8. Take all possible steps to actively discourage the distribution and use of infant-feeding bottles and artificial teats in refugee settings.
9. Advocate that when donations of DSM are supplied to refugee programmes, the specific donors will be approached for cash contributions to be specially earmarked for operational costs of projects to ensure the safe use of this commodity.

Basic principles for the preparation of safe food for infants and young children[1]

Cook food thoroughly

Many raw foods, notably poultry, raw milk, and vegetables, are very often contaminated with disease-causing organisms. Thorough cooking will kill these organisms. For this purpose, all parts of the food must become steaming hot, which means they must reach a minimum temperature of 70 °C.

Avoid storing cooked food

Prepare food for infants and young children freshly, and give it to them immediately after preparation when it is cool enough to eat. Foods prepared for infants and young children should preferably not be stored at all. If this is impossible, food could be stored only for the next meal, but kept cool (at temperatures below 10 °C) or hot (at temperatures near or above 60 °C). Stored food should be reheated thoroughly. Again, this means that all parts of the food must reach at least 70 °C.

[1] Adapted from "Golden rules for safe food preparation" in: *Health surveillance and management procedures for food-handling personnel. Report of a WHO Consultation*, Geneva, World Health Organization, 1989 (WHO Technical Report Series, No. 785), and Basic principles for the preparation of safe food for infants and young children. *Facts about infant feeding*, No. 3, April 1993.

Avoid contact between raw foodstuffs and cooked foods

Cooked food can become contaminated through even the slightest contact with raw food. This cross-contamination can be direct, as, for example, when raw food touches cooked food. It can also be indirect and subtle: for example, through hands, flies, utensils, or unclean surfaces. Thus, hands should be washed after handling high-risk foods, e.g. poultry. Similarly, utensils used for raw foods should be carefully washed before they are used again for cooked food. Dish cloths and hand towels should be washed frequently. The addition of any new ingredients to cooked food may again introduce pathogenic organisms. In this case, food needs to be thoroughly cooked again.

Wash fruits and vegetables

Fruits and vegetables, particularly if they are given to infants in raw form, must be washed carefully with safe water. If possible, they should be peeled immediately before feeding. In situations when these foods are likely to be heavily contaminated, for example when untreated wastewater is used for irrigation or untreated nightsoil is used for soil fertilization, fruits and vegetables that cannot be peeled should be thoroughly cooked before they are given to infants.

Use safe water

Safe water is just as important in preparing food for infants and young children as it is for drinking. Water used in preparing food should be boiled, unless the food to which the water is added has subsequently to be cooked (e.g. rice, potatoes). Ice made with unsafe water will also be unsafe.

Wash hands repeatedly

Wash hands thoroughly before you start preparing or serving food and after every interruption — especially if you have changed the baby's nappy (diaper), used the toilet, or been in contact with animals. It should be remembered that household animals often harbour germs that can pass from hands to food.

Avoid feeding infants with a bottle

Use a cup to give drinks and liquid foods to infants and young children. It is usually difficult to get bottles and teats completely clean. Spoons, cups, dishes, and utensils used for preparing and feeding infants should be washed immediately after use; this will facilitate their thorough cleaning. If bottles and teats must be used, they should be thoroughly washed and boiled after every use.

Protect foods from insects, rodents, and other animals

Animals frequently carry pathogenic organisms and are potential sources of contamination of food.

Store non-perishable foodstuffs in a safe place

Keep pesticides, disinfecting agents, or other toxic chemicals in labelled containers and separate from foodstuffs. To protect against rodents and insects, non-perishable foodstuffs should be stored in closed containers. Containers that have previously held toxic chemicals should not be used for storing foodstuffs.

Keep all food preparation premises meticulously clean

Surfaces used for food preparation must be kept absolutely clean in order to avoid food contamination. Scraps of food and crumbs are potential reservoirs of germs and can attract insects and animals. Garbage should be kept in safe, covered places and be disposed of quickly.

ANNEX 6

Guiding principles for feeding infants and young children in emergencies

Increased mortality and morbidity in emergencies are most serious and most frequent in children under 5 years of age; the increased rates may be as much as 20 times higher than the usual level. This is partly the result of increased exposure to infections, but also due in large measure to inadequate feeding of infants and young children. In recent years awareness of this problem has grown enormously, both as a critical issue for survival of young children and as an aspect of management of nutrition in emergencies. The 10 guiding principles outlined in this annex have been elaborated by WHO to help promote more effective action. More details will be available in:

- *Guiding principles for feeding infants and young children during emergencies.* Geneva, World Health Organization (document in preparation; will be available from Programme of Nutrition, World Health Organization, 1211 Geneva 27, Switzerland).

Full and exclusive breast-feeding of infants until 4–6 months of age is a critical element of optimal feeding, and breast-feeding should continue, with adequate complementary feeding, through to age 2 years if possible. High priority in emergency situations should therefore be given to the following:

- protecting and promoting breast-feeding;
- ensuring provision to, and consumption by, the infant and the lactating mother of adequate energy and nutrient supplies;
- promoting the physical, mental, and social well-being of care-givers;
- ensuring that breast-milk substitutes are used only where they are critically needed, and that safety precautions are observed;
- identifying and eliminating the underlying causes of suboptimal feeding practices.

Breast-feeding

Even in communities where breast-feeding is almost universal, breast-feeding patterns are often undermined in emergencies by the breakdown of traditional care networks. However, shortage of resources and difficulties in safe food preparation for infants make the protection of breast-feeding even more important.

Principle 1. Infants born into populations affected by emergencies should normally be breast-fed.

Breast milk is vital to the growth and development of children during the first months of life. It provides valuable protection against many infections. The first months of breast-feeding favour contraception.

Principle 2. Every effort should be made to create and sustain an environment that encourages frequent breast-feeding of all children under 2 years of age.

Where breast-feeding has been interrupted or mothers are missing or totally unable to breast-feed, strenuous efforts should be made to promote relactation or wet nursing. An appropriate individual should be given full-time responsibility for this. Success hinges on positive development of a woman's attitude, knowledge, and self-confidence, and on frequent suckling. Breast-feeding is the most crucial life-saving activity and should be vigorously supported by health workers and community networks.

Breast-milk substitutes

Principle 3. The quantity, distribution, and use of breast-milk substitutes at emergency sites should be strictly controlled.

Emergency situations tend to aggravate health risks associated with artificial feeding. It should be avoided by raising public awareness through:

- mass media information in donor countries;
- appropriate training of relief programme planners and field staff;
- ensuring that governments and agencies involved in donor and recipient countries are properly informed;
- refusing well-meant but ill-advised donations of "baby foods".

Breast-milk substitutes, fed by cup, should be available only for infants under 6 months of age for whom breast-feeding is not possible and breast milk is not available. For populations that lack a breast-feeding tradition, wider distribution of breast-milk substitutes may be required initially but should be phased out within 6 months by vigorous promotion of breast-feeding among all women who give birth subsequently.

Individuals using breast-milk substitutes should be adequately informed and equipped to ensure their safe and appropriate preparation and use.

Use of breast-milk substitutes in a minority of cases should in no way interfere with protecting and promoting breast-feeding among the majority.

The use of infant-feeding bottles and artificial teats should be actively discouraged.

Complementary feeding

Principle 4. To sustain growth, development and good health, older infants and young children need hygienically prepared foods that are

both easy to eat and digest and that nutritionally complement breast milk.

Complementary foods are usually introduced at 4–6 months of age. In emergencies complementary foods are often coarse, difficult to prepare in soft form, of low nutrient density, and liable to contamination. Their introduction should be delayed until absolutely essential.

The first food is usually a porridge made from a cereal provided in the basic food ration, often together with a pulse, vegetable oil, and vegetables or sugar as available. Suitable locally adapted and feasible recipes and preparation techniques should be worked out and promoted, with special attention to newly responsible caregivers.

Frequent feeding (4–6 times daily) should be encouraged by the provision of fuel and appropriate cooking pots, by using snacks and jointly or collectively prepared meals, and by income-generating activities that allow the purchase of additional foods. Special care is needed to promote appetite, eliminate inhibiting factors, and encourage interaction between child and care-giver.

The complementary foods used should be concentrated sources of dietary energy; special attention should be given to the content of protein, iron, and vitamins A and C. A common problem is that foods provided are too dilute or too bulky.

Principle 5. Caregivers need uninterrupted access to appropriate ingredients with which to prepare nutrient-dense foods for feeding to older infants and young children.

Care-givers' access to essential ingredients can be ensured if:

- food aid and its distribution are well planned;
- local markets are within reach, functioning, and adequately supplied;
- good relations are maintained with local food suppliers;
- income-generating activities and/or household gardening and small-scale animal husbandry are undertaken.

Adequate feeding of infants and young children can be assured only if basic household needs are met. This calls for continuous monitoring of food distribution, household food reserves, and preparation, to identify "food insecure" households.

The contents of the food basket (supplemented from any available resources) should be adequate in amount, taking into account supplies to which people already have access. The commodities should be nutritionally balanced, regularly available, safe for consumption, easy to cook, digestible, and culturally appropriate. They should be equitably distributed among families within the community and in accordance with family size. Families should also know how to distribute equitably according to individual needs — remembering that young children need about 2.5 times as much for size (i.e. per kg of body weight) as adults, and bearing in mind the extra requirements of pregnancy and lactation.

For infants and young children there are special concerns for energy density and micronutrients. Up to now, deficiencies of the latter have been relatively common.

Rations are generally based on cereals, usually with added pulses and oil, and sometimes with sugar and blended foods (cereal–pulse mixes). These foods are commonly rather low in absorbable iron and in vitamins A and C.

Blended foods, especially if fortified, are useful particularly for vulnerable groups. However, provision of blended foods should not be allowed to reduce efforts to promote full use of local products for preparing complementary foods for older infants and young children.

Special commodities sometimes include fresh fruits, vegetables, meat, and fish. Where there is evidence of inadequate intake of essential nutrients, such foods can prevent micronutrient deficiencies.

Selective food distribution for vulnerable groups such as young children may be needed as a temporary measure but the aim is to establish quickly a basic ration adequate to cover the needs of everyone.

Foods available from other sources include the following:

- household food production (e.g. in home or collective gardens) — land must be available, and it may be necessary to supply planting materials, tools, fertilizers, and pesticides;
- foods purchased or bartered, in the market or with neighbours — the relative costs of nutrients obtained in this way should be analysed and explained; various options for increasing income should be explored;
- natural foods that may be available (wild) in the environment — these are usually very nutritious.

Complementary foods should be prepared frequently, safely, and in a clean environment. The basic principles of safe food preparation are detailed in Annex 5.

Caring for care-givers

Principle 6. Because the number of care-givers is reduced during emergencies and their ability to cope is diminished by physical and mental stress, strengthening care-giving capacity is an essential part of promoting good feeding practices for infants and young children.

The physical care of care-givers should include safety, health care, and adequate nutrition. Attention should be paid to the additional food needs of pregnant and lactating women, including wet nurses. In the context of emotional and social security, victims of trauma or rape and the bereaved will have special needs.

Households with only one adult need special attention because of limitations in their mobility, income, self-supporting status, and ability to provide shelter and physical and material security. Opportunities for cooperative child care, income-generation, skills training, etc. should be provided.

Protecting children

Principle 7. To encourage adequate food intake, the health and vigour of children, especially newborns, should be actively protected. Children need to suckle frequently and well, and, as appropriate, to maintain their appetite for complementary foods.

Prenatal care for mothers should include energy and iron supplements, plus iodine and vitamin A in areas where deficiencies of these micronutrients are prevalent.

Appropriate measures to provide protection from illness include promotion of breast-feeding, immunization, environmental health and vector control, and rapid and adequate curative care. Protection from the effects of exposure requires adequate shelter and clothing, especially for newborns.

Infants who are not breast-fed need special care in all these areas because they are highly vulnerable.

Malnutrition

Principle 8. There should be a continual search for malnourished children so that their condition can be identified and treated before it becomes severe. The underlying causes of malnutrition should be investigated and corrected.

Care-givers and community workers should be able to recognize faulty feeding practices, and early symptoms, signs, and probable main causes of malnutrition, and to refer and follow-up recognized cases.

Therapeutic feeding is essential for severely malnourished children, either in hospitals or nutrition rehabilitation centres (which are usually needed if the prevalence of malnutrition exceeds about 10%). Essential elements of management include maintenance of breast-feeding, frequent feeding (initially with a specially formulated liquid diet), and control of infections and fever.

Acute phases of emergencies

Principle 9. To minimize the negative impact of emergencies on feeding practices, interventions should begin immediately, during the acute phase. The focus should be on alleviating pressures on care-givers and channelling scarce resources to meet the nutritional needs of infants and young children.

Appropriate interventions in the acute phase of an emergency would include the following:

- identification of households with infants, young children, and pregnant women, and of the most vulnerable households in this group (e.g. single-parent households, households headed by the elderly, disabled members, etc.);
- priority allocation of resources to these households;
- support for breast-feeding women;

- emergency nourishment for infants whose mothers are absent;
- immediate provision of appropriate emergency foods for feeding young children;
- drawing up locally adapted guidelines for feeding infants and young children;
- developing information/education/communication and feedback systems for young child feeding.

Assessment, intervention and monitoring

Principle 10. Emergencies, by definition, are marked by frequent and rapid change. Promoting optimal feeding for infants and young children in such circumstances requires a flexible approach based on careful continual monitoring.

Assessment priorities for monitoring child-feeding practices include the following:

- dialogue with care-givers to identify current (and desired) feeding practices;
- identification of less appropriate practices and the groups in which they occur;
- identification of decision-makers concerned with infant and young child feeding;
- identification of imperative "quick-fix" measures;
- initial and periodical subsequent gathering of information on
  - — general health and nutritional status
  - — food availability, costs, preparation methods
  - — community attitudes to breast-feeding, relactation, wet nursing, breast-milk substitutes
  - — availability of human resources
  - — income-generating opportunities
  - — services and resources suitable for implementing needed measures.

Essential interventions include the following:

- education and information;
- provision of necessary material resources;
- establishment of communications and support networks;
- coordination with related services;
- development of special programmes for breast-feeding, rehabilitation, orphans.

Effective action depends on setting priorities, searching for solutions, and sustaining the selected action:

- expand and promote existing good practices, curb harmful ones;

- emphasize immediately feasible and sustainable actions that give maximum and lasting results;
- build the capacities of households and communities;
- avoid dependence on single products, e.g. blended foods;
- define objectives and develop a "miniplan" of action for each intervention;
- monitor, using well-defined methods and criteria:
  - — nutritional status of children under 3 years of age and pregnant/lactating women
  - — prevalence of low birth weight
  - — feeding practices (prevalence of exclusive and non-exclusive breast-feeding; adequacy, energy density, frequency, micronutrient content, safety of complementary feeding)
  - — household food security
  - — mortality rates (infants, young children, maternal);
- review activities and refine, enhance, reduce, or replace them as necessary;
- modify action plan accordingly.

Ten steps to successful breast-feeding[1]

Every facility providing maternity services and care for newborn infants should:

1. Have a written breast-feeding policy that is routinely communicated to all health care staff.
2. Train all health care staff in skills necessary to implement this policy.
3. Inform all pregnant women about the benefits and management of breast-feeding.
4. Help mothers initiate breast-feeding within a half-hour of birth.
5. Show mothers how to breast-feed, and how to maintain lactation even if they should be separated from their infants.
6. Give newborn infants no food or drink other than breast milk, unless *medically* indicated.
7. Practise rooming-in — allow mothers and infants to remain together — 24 hours a day.
8. Encourage breast-feeding on demand.
9. Give no artificial teats or pacifiers (also called dummies or soothers) to breast-feeding infants.
10. Foster the establishment of breast-feeding support groups and refer mothers to them on discharge from the hospital or clinic.

[1] From: *Protecting, promoting and supporting breast-feeding: the special role of maternity services.* A joint WHO/UNICEF statement. Geneva, World Health Organization, 1989.

Acceptable medical reasons for using breast-milk substitutes[1]

A few medical indications in a maternity facility may require that individual infants be given fluids or food in addition to, or in place of, breast milk.

It is assumed that severely ill babies, babies in need of surgery, and very low-birth-weight babies (less than 1500g) will be in a special-care unit. Their feeding will be individually decided, given their particular nutritional requirements and functional capabilities, though breast milk is recommended whenever possible. These infants in special care are likely to include:

- infants with very low birth weight or who are born pre-term, at less than 1500g or 32 weeks gestational age;
- severely premature infants with potentially severe hypoglycaemia, or who require therapy for hypoglycaemia, and who do not improve through increased breast-feeding or by being given breast milk.

For babies who are well enough to be with their mothers on the maternity ward, there are very few indications for supplements. In order to assess whether a facility is inappropriately using fluids or breast-milk substitutes, any infants receiving additional supplements must have been diagnosed as:

- infants whose mothers have severe maternal illness (e.g. psychosis, eclampsia, or shock);
- infants with inborn errors of metabolism (e.g. galactosaemia, maple syrup urine disease);
- infants with acute water loss, for example during phototherapy for jaundice, whenever increased breast-feeding cannot provide adequate hydration;
- infants whose mothers are taking medication which is contraindicated when breast-feeding (e.g. cytotoxic drugs, radioactive drugs, and anti-thyroid drugs other than propylthiouracil).

When breast-feeding has to be temporarily delayed or interrupted, mothers should be helped to establish or maintain lactation, for example through manual or hand-pump expression of milk, in preparation for the moment when breast-feeding may be begun or resumed.

HIV and infant feeding: WHO/UNAIDS/UNICEF guidelines

Introduction

The number of infants born with HIV infection is growing every day. The AIDS pandemic represents a tragic setback in the progress made on child welfare and survival.

Given the vital importance of breast milk and breast-feeding for child health, the increasing prevalence of HIV infection around the world, and the evidence of

[1] Reproduced from *WHO/UNICEF Guidelines for the Baby-friendly Hospital Initiative, Part II: Hospital-level implementation*. Geneva, World Health Organization/United Nations Children's Fund, 1992. For a fuller discussion of these and related issues see: Akré J. ed., Infant feeding: the physiological basis, *Bulletin of the World Health Organization*, 1990, 67 (Suppl.).

a risk of HIV transmission through breast-feeding, it is now crucial that policies be developed on HIV infection and infant feeding.

In 1997, the Joint United Nations Programme on HIV/AIDS (UNAIDS) and two of the six co-sponsoring agencies — WHO and UNICEF — issued a joint policy statement on HIV and infant feeding,[1] and initiated the development of guidelines to help national authorities to implement the policy. Other documents on related topics have since been prepared.[2] At the Technical Consultation on HIV and Infant Feeding held in Geneva on 20–22 April 1998, implementation of the guidelines contained in these documents was discussed, and a broad consensus on a public health approach, based on universally recognized human rights standards, has been reached.

The guidelines recognize that:

- HIV infection can be transmitted through breast-feeding. Appropriate alternative to breast-feeding should be available and affordable in adequate amounts for women who have been tested and found to be HIV-positive.
- Breast-feeding is the ideal way to feed the majority of infants. Efforts to protect, promote, and support breast-feeding by women who are HIV-negative or of unknown HIV status need to be strengthened.
- HIV-positive mothers should be enabled to make fully informed decisions about the best way to feed their infants in their particular circumstances. Whatever they decide, they should receive educational, psychosocial, and material support to carry out their decision as safely as possible, including access to adequate alternatives to breast-feeding if they so choose.
- To make fully informed decisions about infant feeding, as well as about other aspects of HIV, mother-to-child transmission, and reproductive life, women need to know and accept their HIV status. There is thus an urgent need to increase access to voluntary and confidential counselling and HIV testing, and to promote its use by women and, when possible, their partners, before alternatives to breast-feeding are made available.
- An essential priority is primary prevention of HIV infection. Education for all adults of reproductive age, particularly for pregnant and lactating women and their sexual partners, and for young people, needs to be strengthened.

Alternative to breast-feeding for HIV-infected mothers

The guidelines describe a number of infant feeding options that women who are HIV-positive may consider, including replacement feeding, modified breast-feeding, and use of breast milk from other sources.

---

[1] *HIV and infant feeding: a policy statement developed collaboratively by UNAIDS, WHO and UNICEF.* Geneva, Joint United Nations Programme on HIV/AIDS, 1997; available from Joint United Nations Programme on HIV/AIDS, 1211 Geneva 27, Switzerland.

[2] *HIV and infant feeding: a review of transmission through breastfeeding.* Geneva, Joint United Nations Programme on HIV/AIDS, 1998 (unpublished document UNAIDS/98.5).
HIV and infant feeding: guidelines for decision makers. Geneva, Joint United Nations Programme on HIV/AIDS, 1998 (unpublished document UNAIDS/98.1).
HIV and infant feeding: a guide for health-care managers and supervisors. Geneva, Joint United Nations Programme on HIV/AIDS, 1998 (unpublished document UNAIDS/98.4). (All available from Joint United Nations Programme on HIV/AIDS, 1211 Geneva 27, Switzerland.)

Replacement feeding means providing a child who receives no breast milk with a diet that contains all the nutrients needed throughout the period for which breast milk is recommended, that is for at least the first 2 years of life.

From birth to 6 months of age, milk is essential and can be given in the form of commercially produced infant formula, or as home-made formula made by modifying fresh or processed animal milk, accompanied by micronutrient supplements (especially iron, zinc, folic acid, and vitamins A and C).

From 6 months to 2 years, replacement feeds should consist of appropriately prepared nutrient-enriched family foods given three times a day if commercial or home-prepared formula continues to be available, or five times a day if neither formula is available. If possible, some form of milk product (such as dried skim milk or yoghurt) should be added to the food as a source of protein and calcium; meat or fish as a source of iron and zinc; and vegetables to provide vitamins A and C, folic acid, and other vitamins. Micronutrient supplements should be given if available.

Families need careful instruction about the preparation of adequate and safe replacement feeds, including accurate mixing, cleaning and sterilizing of utensils, and the use of cups to feed infants instead of bottles. They need resources such as fuel, clean water, and time to enable them to prepare foods safely. The risk of illness and death from replacement feeding must be less than the risk of transmission of HIV through breast-feeding or there will be no advantage in choosing this alternative.

Other options that may be appropriate are modified breast-feeding (early cessation of breast-feeding, or expression and heat treatment of the mother's breast milk), or use of other breast milk (from a breast-milk bank or from an HIV-negative wet-nurse within the family).

Nasogastric tube feeding instructions

Feeding by nasogastric tube is a last-resort emergency procedure that should be carried out only by nurses or other medically trained staff. The procedure is as follows:

- Introduce a moistened tube (internal diameter 2 mm, length 50 cm) into the nose, passing it down the throat and into the stomach. The passage of the tube into the oesophagus is easier if the patient swallows.
- It is essential to check that the tube is in the stomach and not in the lungs. This can be done by using a syringe to remove a small amount of clear fluid from the tube. Alternatively, inject a few ml of air into the tube; if the tube is in the stomach, a loud bubbling noise will be heard in the child's abdomen.
- Secure the tube to the child's temple or cheek with sticking plaster. Carefully check again that the tube is in the stomach. Use a large syringe (50 ml) to feed the normal volume of liquid food slowly down the tube.
- After the feeding, rinse the tube through with a few ml of clean water. It can then be left in place or removed and reinserted at the next feeding.

Nasogastric tubes can also be used to administer oral medicines that cannot be given in any other way.

ANNEX 7

Programme indicators

Indicators of vulnerability and outcome[1]

It has been shown possible on a small scale to build up a coordinated database of information on the nutritional and health circumstances of refugee and displaced populations. A list of possible indicators is given below, but many others could also be included, such as access to fuel, availability of oral rehydration solution, etc. These indicators have been classified as those that reflect or predispose to nutritional and health crises, called vulnerability indicators, and those that measure current nutritional and health problems, called outcome indicators. The latter are dealt with in Chapter 3.

The following two types of vulnerability factor may be identified, although there will inevitably be a degree of overlap:

- "structural risk" factors, such as camp accessibility, which determine long-term vulnerability;
- "process" factors (water supply, market food availability, etc.), which can change rapidly and lead to acute vulnerability.

The building of such a database is intended to:

- identify those camps or population groups in which long-term structural risk factors appear to predispose to nutritional and health crises;
- identify those camps and population groups in which current information on selected process factors indicates a potentially imminent nutritional/health crisis; for example, water supply (expressed as litres per day or number of people per water source) may be an effective predictive indicator;
- improve the overall understanding of factors that predispose to nutritional and health vulnerability among refugees and displaced population groups.

Vulnerability indicators

Structural risk

- Camp isolation/surrounding infrastructures
- Availability of competent supporting agencies
- Season-related factors (epidemics, impassable roads, lack of alternative foods)

[1] Adapted, with permission, from: *Report on testing methods for monitoring the nutrition situation of the refugee and displaced populations.* Geneva, Subcommittee on Nutrition of the United Nations Administrative Committee on Coordination, 1993 (unpublished document).

- Economic assimilation/agricultural self-sufficiency
- Proneness to drought/proximity to civil conflict
- Accuracy of initial registration
- Stability of ecological location
- Endemic disease in area

Process

- Adequacy of water supply
- Market food availability
- Adequacy of health-care provision
- Sanitation
- Immunization coverage
- Food-basket quantity
- Food-basket quality and variety
- Shelter

Outcome indicators

- Prevalence of PEM (usually wasting)
- Prevalence of micronutrient deficiencies
- Mortality
- Morbidity/epidemics

Indicators of the effectiveness of nutritional relief

The purpose of relief programmes in food emergencies is not only to distribute food but also to prevent death and disease and to improve the nutritional status of the affected population. The quantity of food distributed and/or the number of camps or families served are not in themselves adequate measures of the success of a food relief programme. The only acceptable indicators of a programme's success are data indicating positive outcomes in the form of low or decreasing malnutrition levels and death rates.

It is also possible for there to be real improvements that have little or nothing to do with a food relief programme. For example, improvements in climate (and hence agriculture) or other economic conditions may improve and benefit the nutritional status of the population, whether or not the food relief programme is effective.

The indicators discussed in the following paragraphs can be useful in monitoring the effectiveness of a programme.

General feeding programme

Coverage

Comparison of the number of households actually receiving rations with the number entitled to receive them, either from records (if complete) or by sample surveys of households, makes it possible to detect any particular groups that are being excluded.

Adequacy of ration

The adequacy of the ration is usually assessed by "food basket monitoring", in which foods received are compared with the theoretical ration by one of two methods:

- *Exit survey*. Items in hand and the number of persons in the household are checked as people leave a distribution point; the energy value of the food received is calculated per person per day (over the period for which the ration was provided).

More details of food basket monitoring methodology may be found in:
Nutrition guidelines. Paris, Médecins Sans Frontières, 1995.

- *Household survey*. The foods present in a random sample of households are checked on the same day as distribution. However, this method is of limited value because some foods will often have been sold or exchanged already.

Impact

The BMI of adult population samples could be checked periodically. If there has been food shortage, now relieved, BMIs should generally show an upward trend, reaching an adult average of 21–23. Mortality rates should be monitored to identify trends over time.

Selective feeding programme

Coverage

Coverage of the group selected for targeted/selective feeding can be monitored by the following means:

- *Registration.* Comparing the number of children attending relief centres with the number of children in the target population reveals how complete the programme's coverage is. For example:
  - — census data estimate the number of children under 5 years of age as 10 000
  - — camp survey results indicate that 10% of children under 5 years old are more than 2 SD below the median reference weight-for-height
  - — the target population for supplementary feeding should thus be = 0.1 × 10 000 = 1000 children
  - — data from the feeding centre show that 730 children in the target group are actually registered
  - — therefore, the *coverage* of the population at risk = (730/1000) × 100 = 73%.

The above example compares the *projected* size of the population at risk (estimated by the survey) with *actual* registration data for the same target group. It indicates the effectiveness of case-detection for malnourished children, i.e. 73% (assuming an accurate population estimate).

- *Attendance*. The monthly attendance rate of registered children is a helpful measure of the acceptability and accessibility of selective feeding. Continuing the example above:
  - — monthly average number of children *attending* the feeding programme = 500
  - — therefore, percentage of the total registered actually attending = (500/730) × 100 = 69%.

At community level, this indicates whether the programme is accessible and acceptable. Attendance rates also highlight how much follow-up is needed on individual children who are registered but are not attending.

Impact

Weight gain is a critical indicator of programme success or impact, yet undernourished children may gain some weight and still fall into a deficient nutritional category. As part of regular programme monitoring, the following estimates should be made:

- At household/community/health-centre level:
  - — The percentage of children losing weight over a 1-month period (which should be 0).
  - — The percentage of children shifting from one nutritional category to another, such as from between −2SD and −3SD below median reference weight-for-height, either upwards to above −2SD or downwards to below median −3SD, over a given period of time.
- In rehabilitation centres or programmes (e.g. domiciliary rehabilitation or follow-up clinics for children who were severely malnourished):
  - — The average daily weight gain per kg of body weight. The daily weight gain in "normal" reference children between 1 and 5 years old is well under 1g per kg of body weight. In malnourished children, the gain must be much higher to indicate recovery — it should be 10–15g per kg of body weight per day. If oedema was present, the rate of gain should be calculated from the time oedema was lost.
  - — The percentage of children who are responding to treatment over a 1-month period, i.e. the percentage of childen gaining more than 5g per kg of body weight (a minimum acceptable rate).

ANNEX 8

Biochemical assessment of micronutrients

Assessment of thiamine deficiency

The clinical signs of beriberi are described in Chapter 2, but there are several biochemical and other methods that provide a more sensitive assessment of thiamine status. The most common determinations are the following:

- urinary thiamine excretion, per 6- or 24-hour period or per gram of creatinine (see Table A8.1);
- erythrocyte transketolase levels, and the increase that occurs on addition of thiamine pyrophosphate (TPP), expressed as a percentage of the basal level; this increase is termed the thiamine pyrophosphate effect (TPPE) or erythrocyte ketolase activity coefficient (ETK-AC) (see Table A8.2);
- breast-milk thiamine levels, used as a measure of both maternal and infant thiamine status (see Table A8.3);
- thiamine levels in whole blood and in erythrocytes;
- blood pyruvate levels;
- dietary thiamine intake;
- increases in monthly mortality rates among infants aged 2–5 months.

Criteria for assessing the public health significance of thiamine deficiency are summarized in Table A8.4.

Assessment of niacin deficiency

The clinical signs of pellagra are described in Chapter 2, but there are biochemical and other methods that provide a more sensitive assessment of niacin status. The most common determinations are the following:

- urinary excretion of N^1-methylnicotinamide, per 24-hour period or per gram of creatinine (see Table A8.5);
- ratio of niacin metabolites in urine — (6-pyridone):(N^1-methylnicotinamide);
- loading tests with nicotinic acid, nicotinamide, or tryptophan;
- dietary intake of niacin equivalents.

Interpretation of these biochemical parameters is somewhat equivocal, and dietary surveys are difficult to organize. Provisional criteria for assessing the public health significance of niacin deficiency in the absence of other available tests are summarized in Table A8.6.

***Table A8.1** Guidelines for the interpretation of urinary excretion of thiamine*[a]

Parameter	Deficient (high risk)	Low (medium risk)	Acceptable (low risk)
Urinary thiamine (μg/g creatinine)			
Children:			
1–3 years	<120	120–175	176
4–6 years	<85	85–120	121
7–9 years	<70	70–180	181
10–12 years	<60	60–180	181
13–15 years	<50	50–150	151
Adults	<27	27–65	66
Pregnancy			
2nd trimester	<23	23–54	55
3rd trimester	<21	21–49	50
Urinary thiamine (μg)			
Adults			
per 6-hour period	<10	10–24	25
per 24-hour period	<40	40–99	100
Load test (% return of 5-mg thiamine dose in 4-hour period)			
Adults	<20	20–79	80

[a] Adapted, with permission, from: Sauberlich HE, Skala JH, Dowdy RP. *Laboratory tests for the assessment of nutritional status.* Cleveland, OH, CRC Press, 1974.

***Table A8.2** Classification and interpretation of TPPE (thiamine pyrophosphate effect) levels in individuals*[a]

Thiamine status	TPPE (%)
Normal	0–14
Marginally deficient	15–24
Severely deficient (with clinical signs)	≥25

[a] Reproduced, with permission, from: Brin M et al. Some preliminary findings on the nutritional status of the aged in Onondaga county, New York. *American journal of clinical nutrition*, 1965, 17:240–258.

Assessment of ascorbic acid deficiency

The clinical signs of scurvy are described in Chapter 2, but there are several biochemical and other methods that provide a more sensitive assessment of ascorbic acid (vitamin C) status. The most common determinations are the following:

- serum or whole plasma levels of ascorbic acid (see Table A8.7);
- whole blood levels of ascorbic acid (see Table A8.7);
- leukocyte ascorbic acid levels (see Table A8.7);
- urinary excretion of ascorbic acid or ascorbate-2-sulfate, per 24-hour period or per gram of creatinine;
- ascorbic acid saturation or loading tests.

Table A8.3 *Breast-milk thiamine levels: provisional criteria for assessment in individuals*

Thiamine status	Breast-milk thiamine (μg/litre)
Normal	100–200
Marginally deficient	50–99
Severely deficient	<50

Table A8.4 *Provisional criteria for severity of public health problem of thiamine deficiency*

Indicator		Severity of public health problem		
		Mild	Moderate	Severe
Clinical signs		≥1 clinical case; <1% of population in age group concerned	1–4% of population in age group concerned	≥5% of population in age group concerned
TPPE test ≥25%		5–19%	20–49%	≥50%
Urinary thiamine (μg/g creatinine)				
Adults:	% below 27	5–19%	20–49%	≥50%
Children:				
1–3 years	% below 120			
4–6 years	% below 85			
7–9 years	% below 70			
10–12 years	% below 60			
13–15 years	% below 50			
Pregnancy:				
2nd trimester	% below 23			
3rd trimester	% below 21			
Breast-milk thiamine <50 μg/litre		5–19%	20–49%	≥50%
Dietary intake <0.33 mg/1000 $kcal_{th}$		5–19%	20–49%	≥50%
Mortality among infants aged 2–5 months		No decline in rates	Slight peak in rates	Marked peak in rates

Table A8.5 *Guidelines for the interpretation of urinary excretion of niacin metabolites*[a]

Parameter	Deficient	Low	Acceptable	High
Urinary N^1-methylnicotinamide (mg per g creatinine)				
Adults (men; women, non-pregnant or 1st trimester pregnancy)	<0.5	0.5–1.59	1.6–4.29	≥4.3
Pregnant women:				
2nd trimester	<0.6	0.6–1.99	2.0–4.99	≥5.0
3rd trimester	<0.8	0.8–2.49	2.5–6.49	≥6.5
Ratio 2-pyridone:N^1-methylnicotinamide	<0.5	<1.0	1.0–4.0	
Dietary intake of niacin equivalents (mg/day)	<5	5–9	≥10	

[a] Sources:
Sauberlich HE, Skala JH, Dowdy RP. *Laboratory tests for the assessment of nutritional status.* Cleveland, OH, CRC Press, 1974.
Dillon JC et al. Les metabolites urinaires de la niacine au cours de la pellagre. [Urinary metabolites of niacin in pellagra.] *Annals of nutrition and metabolism,*1992, 36:181–185.
Malfait P et al. An outbreak of pellagra related to changes in dietary niacin among Mozambican refugees in Malawi. *International journal of epidemiology,* 1993, 22:504–511.

Table A8.6 *Provisional criteria for severity of public health problem of niacin deficiency*

Indicator	Severity of public health problem		
	Mild	Moderate	Severe
Clinical signs	≥1 clinical case; <1% of population in age group concerned	1–4% of population in age group concerned	≥5% of population in age group concerned
Urinary N^1-methylnicotinamide <0.50 mg per gram creatinine	5–19%	20–49%	≥50%
Ratio 2-pyridone: N^1-methylnicotinamide <1.0	5–19%	20–49%	≥50%
Dietary intake of niacin equivalents <5 mg/day	5–19%	20–49%	≥50%

Table A8.7 *Guidelines for the interpretation of ascorbic acid levels in individuals of all ages*[a]

Indicator	Deficient (high risk)	Low (medium risk)	Acceptable (low risk)
Serum ascorbic acid (mg/100 ml)	<0.20	0.20–0.29	>0.30
Leukocyte ascorbic acid (nmol/10^8 cells)	<57	57–114	>114
Whole blood ascorbic acid[b] (mg/100 ml)	<0.30	0.30–0.49	>0.50

[a] Reproduced, with permission, from: Sauberlich HE, Skala JH, Dowdy RP. *Laboratory tests for the assessment of nutritional status*. Cleveland, OH, CRC Press, 1974. Data kindly updated by Dr H.E. Sauberlich.

[b] This classification may not be valid for individuals with marked anaemia.

Table A8.8 *Provisional criteria for severity of public health problem of ascorbic acid deficiency*[a]

Indicator	Severity of public health problem		
	Mild	Moderate	Severe
Clinical signs	≥1 clinical case; <1% of population in age group concerned	1–4% of population in age group concerned	≥5% of population in age group concerned
Serum ascorbic acid (mg/100 ml):			
<0.20	10–29%	30–49%	≥50%
<0.30	30–49%	50–69%	≥70%

[a] Sources:
Sauberlich HE, Skala JH, Dowdy RP. *Laboratory tests for the assessment of nutritional status*. Cleveland, OH, CRC Press, 1974.
Desenclos JC et al. Epidemiological patterns of scurvy among Ethiopian refugees. *Bulletin of the World Health Organization*, 1989, 67:309–316.

Only the first of these tests is widely used, reliable, and practicable in field surveys. Care must be taken both in conserving serum/plasma samples and to avoid haemolysis (which can lead to false results). Criteria for assessing the public health significance of ascorbic acid deficiency are summarized in Table A8.8.

Summary of laboratory methods and samples required

General principles

Micronutrients are essentially labile or are found in labile compounds, and analysis is technically difficult, both because of this lability and because of the presence in blood, urine, and breast milk of substances that interfere with analysis. Thus, although it is not difficult to specify the analytical method or methods commonly used, great care is required to obtain reliable and accurate results. It would be wise for any laboratory starting up new work in this area to contact a well established facility with experience in the assessment of the nutrient concerned and to carry out a calibration procedure; this should ensure that equivalent and internationally acceptable results are obtained. On request, WHO can provide a list of leading laboratories with experience in the assessment of the various nutrients.[1]

The equipment and reagents required, references to the basic biochemical methods for the assessment of iron, iodine, and vitamin A status, and general requirements for a micronutrient laboratory are detailed in the following publication:

- May WA et al. *Micronutrient laboratory: equipment manual.* Atlanta, GA, Programme against Micronutrient Malnutrition, 1996.

For specific nutrients, a summary of the main methods and references is given in the publications or documents cited in the following paragraphs.

Anaemia and iron status

Assessing anaemia: haemoglobin and haematocrit (erythrocyte volume fraction)

These are two basic and widely used tests for assessing anaemia, which are simple to perform and can provide reasonably good information about iron status. However, the need for proper standardization, supervision, and quality control of these procedures, plus training in their use, should not be overlooked. Various methods are discussed in the following publication:

- *Anemia detection in health services: guidelines for program managers.* Seattle, WA, Program for Appropriate Technology in Health, 1996.

Haemoglobin

The *cyanmethaemoglobin method*[2] is considered to be the most accurate and reliable method of determining haemoglobin. Details are contained in the following publication:

- *Procedure for the quantitative determination of haemoglobin in blood.* Villanova, PA, National Committee for Clinical Laboratory Standards, 1984.

In the field, dried blood spot samples can be used for performing the test. These are prepared by applying a drop of whole blood to a special filter paper, which is

[1] Available on request from Programme of Nutrition, World Health Organization, 1211 Geneva 27, Switzerland.

[2] The method requires a well trained laboratory technician, routine instrument calibration, careful execution, and attention to proper method standardization and quality control practices.

then allowed to dry. Once dried, the samples remain fairly stable, even without freezing. Small battery-operated colorimeters are now available that allow determinations to be made outside a laboratory setting.

A simple, transportable, robust haemoglobin photometer is now available that can be used for accurate haemoglobin testing in the field. It uses disposible sample cuvettes into which blood is drawn, and which are then placed in the instrument for automatic haemoglobin measurement. Results are available in 1–2 minutes and are comparable to laboratory methods in terms of accuracy and precision. The instrument can be used by non-laboratory personnel after minimal training. The high cost of the test cuvettes limits routine use, but the instrument can play a valuable role in rapid nutrition surveys or sentinel site surveillance. The instrument is reviewed in the following publication:

- Johns WL, Lewis SM. Primary health screening by haemoglobinometry in a tropical community. *Bulletin of the World Health Organization*, 1989, 67(6):627–633.

In the *filter-paper method*, a spot of capillary blood is collected directly on filter paper and compared with a printed set of colour standards. This method is inexpensive, simple, portable, and rapid, and therefore useful for screening in rural settings. However, it is highly subjective and inappropriate as a stand-alone test. Recently, WHO has developed a reliable haemoglobin colour scale for use with standard-quality filter paper; its suitability and reliability for use in various field conditions are currently being assessed. Details are given in the following publication:

- Stott GM, Lewis SM. A simple and reliable method for estimating haemoglobin. *Bulletin of the World Health Organization* 1995, 73(3):369–373.

Haematocrit (erythrocyte volume fraction)[1]

Determination of haematocrit can be used as an alternative to haemoglobin testing. The method involves spinning a small volume of blood collected into a heparinized glass capillary tube, using a special microhaematocrit centrifuge. Its advantages are technical simplicity, low operational costs, and the fact that it can be done outside the laboratory. Details are given in the following publication:

- *Procedure for determining packed cell volume by the microhematocrit method*, 2nd ed. Villanova, PA, National Committee for Clinical Laboratory Standards, 1993.

Assessing iron status

Serum ferritin, erythrocyte protoporphyrin, transferrin saturation, transferrin receptors, and red cell indices, especially mean corpuscular volume, provide much more insight into iron status. The tests are more sensitive than those for determining haemoglobin and haematocrit and confirm the presence of underlying iron deficiency. However, because of the cost and the sophistication of these

[1] The method requires a well trained laboratory technician, routine instrument calibration, careful execution, and attention to proper method standardization and quality control practices.

methods, large-scale use is not common; usage is generally limited to special surveys or to settings where resources are relatively abundant.

A general reference on assessment of iron status is:

- *Measurements of iron status.* Washington, DC, International Nutritional Anaemia Consultative Group, 1985.

Serum ferritin

Serum ferritin is the most specific and sensitive biochemical test for iron deficiency; when used in combination with haemoglobin, it may offer the greatest potential for monitoring iron deficiency. However, serum ferritin is often elevated in response to infectious or inflammatory conditions. Methods are detailed in the following publications:

- Miles LEM et al. The measurement of serum ferritin by a 2-site immunoradiometric assay. *Annals of biochemistry*, 1974, 61:209–224. (This is the conventional immunoradiometric assay method.[1])
- Pintar J et al. A screening test for assessing iron status. *Blood*, 1982, 59:110–113. (A semi-quantitative ferritin measurement based on a modification of a two-site enzyme-linked immunoassay. It requires only 2 drops of blood, i.e. 35 μl serum, and a total incubation time of 90 minutes. It can be performed without laboratory facilities and is therefore suitable for use in fieldwork.)
- May WA. *Micronutrient laboratory equipment manual.* Atlanta, GA, Program Against Micronutrient Malnutrition, 1996. (Details are provided for newer non-radioactive enzyme-linked immunoassay.)

Erythrocyte protoporphyrin

Protoporphyrin is a precursor of haem and accumulates in red cells when there is insufficient iron to make haem. Elevated levels occur in the second stage of iron deficiency and after iron stores have been depleted. Erythrocyte protoporphyrin correlates well with low serum ferritin and can serve as a screening test for moderate iron deficiency. However, elevated levels can also be difficult to interpret in areas where infection rates are high. The method is described in the following publication:

- Blumberg WE, Doleiden FH, Lamol AA. Haemoglobin determined in 15 μl of whole blood by "front-face" fluorometry. *Clinical chemistry*, 1980, 26:409–413.

Transferrin saturation

Almost all of the iron in the serum is bound to the iron-binding protein, transferrin. Transferrin saturation is calculated by measuring both serum iron and total iron-binding capacity using spectrophotometric techniques, dividing the iron concentration by the iron-binding capacity, and multiplying the result by 100 to yield a percentage. The method is described in the following publication:

[1] The method requires a well trained laboratory technician, routine instrument calibration, careful execution, and attention to proper method standardization and quality control practices.

- Summary of a report on assessment of the iron nutritional status of the United States population. Expert Scientific Working Group. *American journal of clinical nutrition*, 1985, 42:1318–1330.

Serum transferrin receptors

This newer test for serum transferrin receptors has the advantage of being unaffected by the presence of infection; however, it is affected by any increase in red-cell turnover, e.g. haemolysis. The method is described in the following publication:

- Flowers CH et al. The clinical measurement of serum transferrin receptors. *Journal of laboratory and clinical medicine*, 1988, 114:368–377.

Red cell indices

When measured by electronic blood counters, mean corpuscular volume and red cell distribution width are reliable indices of iron deficiency; the indices are not very sensitive, however, and change only when anaemia is also apparent.

Iodine

Indicators of iodine deficiency are discussed in the following publication:

- *Indicators for assessing iodine deficiency disorders and their control through salt iodization*. Geneva, World Health Organization, 1994 (unpublished document WHO/NUT/94.6).[1]

The main test of thyroid function is the thyroid-stimulating hormone level. Methods are outlined in the following publication:

- May WA. *Micronutrient laboratory: equipment manual*. Atlanta, GA, Program Against Micronutrient Malnutrition, 1996.

Vitamin A

Indicators for assessing vitamin A deficiency are discussed in the following publication:

- *Indicators for assessing vitamin A deficiency and their application in monitoring and evaluating intervention programmes*. Geneva, World Health Organization, 1996 (unpublished document WHO/NUT/96.10).[1]

Thiamine

The most commonly used procedure for assessing thiamine status has been the measurement of erythrocyte transketolase activity and its stimulation *in vitro* by the addition of thiamine pyrophosphate (TPP effect).

The erythrocyte transketolase activity assay involves the incubation of haemolysed whole blood samples in a buffered medium with an excess of ribose-

---

[1] Available on request from Programme of Nutrition, World Health Organization, 1211 Geneva 27, Switzerland.

5-phosphate, in both the presence and absence of excess thiamine pyrophosphate.

Details of the erythrocyte transketolase activity assay are given in the following publications:

- Duffy P, Morris P, Neilson G. Thiamin status of a Melanesian population. *American journal of clinical nutrition*, 1981,343:1584–1592. (Using a bichromatic analyser to provide semiautomated measurement of the stimulation of erythrocyte transketolase by thiamine pyrophosphate.)
- Smeets E, Muller H, de Wael J et al. A NADH-dependent transketolase assay in erythrocyte hemolysates. *Clinica chimica acta*, 1971, 33:379–86. (Manual method for TPP effect.)
- Waring P et al. A continuous-flow (AutoAnalyzer II) procedure for measuring erythrocyte transketolase activity. *Clinical chemistry*, 1982, 28:2206–2213. (Simple, rapid, semiautomated assay for transketolase activity.)
- Bayoumi RA, Rosalki SB. Evaluation of methods of coenzyme activation of erythrocyte enzymes for detection of deficiency of vitamins B1, B2, and B6. *Clinical chemistry*, 1976, 22:327–35. (Ultraviolet spectrophotometric procedure.)
- Basu TK, Patel DR, Williams DC et al. A simplified microassay of transketolase in human blood. *International journal for vitamin and nutrition research*, 1974, 44:319–326. (Calorimetric method.)
- Kimura M, Itokawa Y. Determination of blood transketolase by high-performance liquid chromatography. *Journal of chromatography*, 1982, 239:707–710. (Measures the amount of transketolase present rather than the enzyme activity. A micromethod that requires further development and validation.)
- Vuilleumier JP, Keller HE, Keck E. Clinical chemical methods for the routine assessment of the vitamin status in human populations. Part III: The apoenzyme stimulation tests for vitamin B1, B2 and B6 adapted to the Cobas-Bio analyzer. *International journal for vitamin and nutrition research*, 1989, 60:126–135. (Assay using centrifugal analyser.)

The following publications provide details of the determination of thiamine in blood:

- Fidanza F. *Nutritional assessment: a manual for population studies.* London, Chapman & Hall, 1991.
- Tietz NW. *Clinical guide to laboratory tests*, 3rd ed. Philadelphia, W.B. Saunders, 1995.
- Finglas PM. Thiamin. *International journal for vitamin and nutrition research*, 1993, 63:270–274.

The following publications provide details of the determination of thiamine in urine:

- Roser RL et al. Determination of urinary thiamin by high-pressure liquid chromatography utilizing the thiochrome fluorescent method. *Journal of chromatography*, 1978, 146:43–53.
(Method comparable to using the microbiological assay.)

- Dong MH, Green MD, Sauberlich HE. Determination of urinary thiamin by the thiochrome method. *Clinical biochemistry*, 1981, 14:16–18.
- Pearson W. Biochemical appraisal of nutritional status in man. *American journal of clinical nutrition*, 1962, 11:462–476.
- O'Neal RM, Johnson OC, Schaefer AE. Guidelines for classification and interpretation of group blood and urine data collected as part of the National Nutrition Survey. *Pediatric research*, 1970, 4:103–106.
- Hennessy DJ, Cerecedo LR. Determination of free phosphorylated thiamin by a modified thiochrome assay. *Journal of the American Chemical Society*, 1939, 61:179–183.
- Nail PA, Thomas MR, Eakin R. The effect of thiamin and riboflavin supplementation on the level of those vitamins in human breast milk and urine. *American journal of clinical nutrition*, 1980, 33:198–204.

Methods for the determination of thiamine in breast milk are detailed in the following publications:

- Kendall N. Thiamin content of various milks. *Journal of pediatrics*, 1942, 20:65–73. (The thiochrome method.)
- Valyasevi A et al. Chemical compositions of breast milk in different locations of Thailand. *Journal of the Medical Association of Thailand*, 1968, 51:348–353.
- Hennessy DJ et al. Determination of free phosphorylated thiamin by a modified thiochrome assay. *Journal of the American Chemical Society*, 1939, 61:179–183. (Standard method of the Infant Formula Council.)
- Nail PA, Thomas MR, Eakin R. The effect of thiamin and riboflavin supplementation on the level of those vitamins in human breast milk and urine. *American journal of clinical nutrition*, 1980, 33:198–204.

Niacin

Only a few laboratory procedures are available for assessing niacin status. The general procedure is to measure one or more urinary excretion products of niacin metabolism, most commonly N^1-methylnicotinamide (N^1-MN) and 2-pyridone. The excretion ratio of 2-pyridone to N^1-MN is the most reliable indicator of niacin nutritional status. More recently, high-pressure liquid chromatography techniques have been applied to plasma and urine samples to measure nicotinic acid, nicotinamide, and their metabolites. There have been reports on the use of modified microbiological assay procedures for determining the biologically active forms of niacin in plasma and blood. For laboratories lacking appropriate chromatography equipment, an extremely sensitive fluorometric procedure has been reported for the measurement of N^1-MN and nicotinamide in serum.

In practice, laboratory assessment of niacin nutritional status is still limited to the measurement of niacin metabolites in urine. The availability of high-pressure liquid chromatography simplifies the process and enhances the speed, accuracy, and sensitivity of determinations of 2-pyridone and N^1-MN in urine. General reference to determination of niacin may be found in the following publication:

- Sauberlich HE. Newer laboratory methods for assessing nutriture of selected B-complex vitamins. *Annual reviews of nutrition*, 1984, 4:377–407.

Methods for assessing niacin nutritional status using urine samples is detailed in the following publications:

- Goldsmith GA et al. Studies of niacin requirement in man. I. Experimental pellagra in subjects on corn diets low in niacin and tryptophan. *Journal of clinical investigation*, 1952, 31:533–542. (Microbiological methods for the determination of niacin and tryptophan and fluorometric methods for the determination of N^1-MN and 6-pyridone.)
- Dillon JC et al. Les metabolites urinaires de la niacine au cours de la pellagre. [Urinary metabolites of niacin in pellagra.] *Annals of nutrition and metabolism*, 1992, 36:181–185. (High-pressure liquid chromatography method for measuring excretion ratio of 2-pyridone to N^1-MN.)

Methods for assessing niacin nutritional status using plasma and blood samples are described in the following publications:

- Gravesen J. pH metric method for the determination of nicotinic acid in plasma. *Journal of clinical microbiology*, 1977, 5:390–392. (Microbiological assay procedure for determination of the biologically active forms of niacin in plasma and blood.)
- Kertcher JA et al. A radiometric microbiologic assay for the biologically active forms of niacin. *Journal of nuclear medicine*, 1979, 20:419–423. (Radiometric microbiological assay requiring use of tracer amounts of a radioisotope.)

Ascorbic acid

The measurement of serum levels of ascorbic acid is the most commonly used and practical procedure for evaluating vitamin C nutritional status in population groups or individuals. White blood cell levels of ascorbic acid provide information concerning the body stores of the vitamin, but the measurement is technically difficult to perform and its use is confined to clinical situations as an aid in the diagnosis of scurvy. Information on urinary levels of ascorbic acid and the use of vitamin C loading tests can also be helpful in the clinical diagnosis of scurvy.

Assessment of vitamin C status using serum, blood, or urine samples is described in the following publications:

- Schaffert RR, Kingsley GR. A rapid, simple method for the determination of reduced, dehydro-, and total ascorbic acid in biological material. *Journal of biological chemistry*, 1955, 212:59. (Using either dinitrophenylhydrazine or 2,6-dichloroindophenol reagent.)
- Deutsch MJ, Weeks CE. Microfluorimetric assay for vitamin C. *Journal — Association of Official Analytical Chemists*, 1965, 48:1248–1256. (Method shows a high degree of specificity.)

The following publication describes the assessment of vitamin C status using urine samples:

- March SC. A quantitative procedure for the assay of ascorbate-3-sulfate in biological samples. *Federation proceedings*, 1972, 31: 705.

Assessment of vitamin C status using serum/plasma samples is detailed in the following publications:

- Goad WC et al. *A semiautomated technique for the determination of vitamin C in serum or plasma samples*. US Army Medical Research and Nutrition Laboratory Report, Denver, CO, June 1972.
- Brubacher G, Vuilleumier JP, Vitamin C. In: Curtis HC, Roth M, eds. *Clinical biochemistry — principles and methods*. Berlin, Walter de Gruyter, 1974.
- Bates CJ. Plasma vitamin C assays: a European experience. *International journal for vitamin and nutrition research*, 1994, 64:283–287.

ANNEX 9

Human resource development for the management of nutrition in major emergencies: outline of an educational programme

This manual deals with planning and management of the nutrition component of preparedness for and response to major emergencies. Its essential purpose is to help build national capacity for these activities, and this necessarily implies human resource development within the country concerned. This annex provides a framework for an educational programme in this area, in the form of appropriate general, intermediate, and specific objectives. These objectives are based on the problems likely to be encountered; they would naturally have to be adapted to national circumstances, as would the specific content of the educational programme.

In practice, a core of national personnel is likely to be called upon to organize short-term training of key individuals in the management of nutrition in emergencies. If a national-level training team is not yet available, the initial training workshop should be of the nature of a "training of trainers". Such training would normally proceed in "cascade" fashion. That is, it would be provided initially for personnel at national level — particularly those in charge of primary health care, maternal and child health, and nutrition and food safety and disease control programmes, probably together with regional/provincial health directors from disaster-prone areas of the country. Subsequently, the training would take place at the regional/provincial level for other personnel at that level, together with key individuals from the district health team (district health officer, and those responsible for mother and child health, nutrition, nursing, environmental health, etc.). Later, there should be training for key personnel from each health centre or sub-centre at the district level (or from at-risk areas within the district).

Finally, there should be some orientation of community health workers, health committees, etc., at village level on appropriate community action to ensure adequate and optimum nutrition (within the constraints of the situation and available resources).

The objectives outlined in Tables A9.1 and A9.2 cover the essential requirements at national level. Appropriate amendment and simplification would be necessary to adapt them to the activities to be carried out at subsequent — lower — levels.

Examples of learning materials are being developed globally for use in initial interregional training programmes, but the development of nationally and locally appropriate learning materials, suitable for the local situation and the educational background of the personnel concerned, is preferable.

In addition to organizing in-service training of existing personnel, all emergency-prone countries should ideally review the basic curricula in schools of health

Table A9.1 *Overall objectives of training in emergencies*

General objectives	Intermediate objectives
The programme should enable national programme managers and related personnel in national emergency preparedness and response programmes who follow the course to:	
1. Identify populations at nutritional risk in emergency situations	1.1 Establish that a nutritional emergency or risk exists 1.2 Quantify the main nutritional problems present or likely to occur 1.3 Identify the main causal factors
2. Determine the food resources available	2.1 Determine where there is inadequate (in quality or quantity) food availability or access, affecting the whole population or selected groups 2.2 Identify particularly vulnerable groups (physiological, geographical, socioeconomic)
3. Estimate the nutritional, food and related requirements of affected and at-risk populations	3.1 Plan what food distribution is needed, and appropriate rations and other interventions 3.2 Ensure optimal general care of vulnerable groups, especially mothers and young children
4. Manage severe malnutrition and related illness in the affected populations	4.1 Organize appropriate nutritional rehabilitation of severely malnourished individuals 4.2 Ensure appropriate management of intercurrent infections
5. Ensure effective integration of nutrition in primary health care for at-risk populations	5.1 Identify relevant available preventive health services and primary health care (community-based) programmes, the response capacity, and where they need strengthening 5.2 Assess the adequacy of nutrition, food safety and food aid components of these activities, the response capacity, and where they need strengthening
6. Plan and implement a human resource development programme in the management of and preparedness for nutritional emergencies (in the trainee's own country)	6.1 Identify appropriate personnel for training at each administrative level 6.2 Plan and implement an educational programme for the management of nutrition in emergencies
7. Evaluate the nutrition-in-emergency programme	7.1 Design a monitoring and evaluation system for the programme of response and preparedness for nutrition in major emergencies: (a) process and outcomes (b) impact

Table A9.2 *Specific objectives of training in emergencies*

Intermediate objective	Specific objectives
1. Identify populations at nutritional risk in emergency situations	
1.1 Establish that a nutritional emergency or risk exists	1.1.1 Carry out rapid assessment; collect existing information; rapid survey if needed in limited area 1.1.2 Identify and analyse indicators of nutritional emergency and of nutritional risk (early warning system)
1.2 Quantify the main nutritional problems present or likely to occur	1.2.1 Estimate prevalence of main nutritional disorders (PEM, anaemia, iodine and vitamin deficiencies) in a valid statistical sample of children <5 years and in a subsample of adults (men and women) 1.2.2 Identify the main geographical and socio-economic groups at risk or affected 1.2.3 Assess infant, young child, and overall mortality in affected populations
1.3 Identify the main causal factors	1.3.1 Assess the main causes (relating to food, health, and care)

Table A9.2 *(continued)*

Intermediate objective	Specific objectives
2. Determine the food resources available	
2.1 Determine where there is inadequate (in quality or quantity) food availability or access, affecting the whole population	2.1.1 Collect and analyse information on overall food supplies and availability in the at-risk area (per head), including local production potential, market supplies, and food aid "in the pipeline"
2.2 Identify particular groups (physiological, geographical, socio-economic) affected or at risk	2.2.1 Collect and analyse information on food consumption patterns, and access to food by category of household, geographical, and socio-economic group 2.2.2 Assess the adequacy of consumption by each group
3. Estimate the nutritional, food, and related requirements of affected/at-risk populations	
3.1 Plan what food distribution is needed, and appropriate rations	3.1.1 Calculate energy and nutrient requirements for target populations 3.1.2 Plan appropriate nutrient requirements and food rations for generalized food distribution and targeted supplementary feeding 3.1.3 Establish criteria for each of these types of intervention
3.2 Ensure optimal care of vulnerable groups, especially mothers and young children	3.2.1 Establish guidelines for appropriate general care and support of mothers, newborns, infants, and young children
4. Manage severe malnutrition and related illnesses in affected populations	
4.1 Organize appropriate nutritional rehabilitation of severely malnourished individuals	4.1.1 Establish nutritional rehabilitation wards or centres; ensure adequate staffing and equipment 4.1.2 Establish (or use existing) practical guidelines for routine management of PEM and micronutrient deficiencies 4.1.3 Identify current wrong practices
4.2 Ensure appropriate management of intercurrent infections	4.2.1 Establish (or use existing) guidelines for prevention and treatment of common intercurrent infections
5. Ensure effective integration of nutrition in primary health care for at-risk populations	
5.1 Identify relevant available preventive health services and primary health care (community- based) programmes, the response capacity, and where they need strengthening	5.1.1 Assess functional adequacy of main relevant preventive services, especially prevention and surveillance of infectious diseases, and corresponding community-based action 5.1.2 Make recommendations for strengthening these services
5.2 Assess the adequacy of nutrition, food safety, and food aid components, the response capacity, and where these need strengthening	5.2.1 Assess functional adequacy of nutrition, food safety, and food aid components 5.2.2 Make recommendations for strengthening these components
6. Plan a human resource development programme in the management of and preparedness for nutrition in emergencies	
6.1 Identify appropriate personnel for training at each administrative level	6.1.1 Define appropriate elements of job descriptions for various categories of personnel involved in the management of nutrition in emergencies, relating to nutrition, food safety, and food aid

Table A9.2 *(continued)*

Intermediate objective	Specific objectives
6.2 Plan and implement an educational programme for the management of nutrition in emergencies	6.2.1 Define educational objectives, adapted to local needs 6.2.2 Define essential course content and learning materials needed 6.2.3 Develop appropriate examination instruments
7. Evaluate the nutrition in emergencies programme	
7.1 Design a monitoring and evaluation system for the nutrition in emergencies programme as a whole (a) Process	7.1.1 Define process indicators (relevance, progress, effectiveness) and criteria of adequacy of each programme component and of the programme as a whole 7.1.2 Define procedures for monitoring and evaluating the programme
7.2 As 7.1 (b) Impact	7.2.1 Define impact indicators and criteria of adequacy of each programme component and of the programme as a whole 7.2.2 Define procedures for monitoring and evaluating the programme

sciences (as they relate to emergency-preparedness and response, and nutrition) to ensure incorporation of appropriate subject matter.

Details of these processes are beyond the scope of this manual, but the interested reader is referred to: Oshaug A, Benbouzid D, Guilbert J-J. *Educational handbook for nutrition trainers: how to increase your skills and make it easier for students to learn.* Geneva, World Health Organization, 1993.